Calculations and Constants
for
Clinical Practice

Calculations and Constants
for
Clinical Practice

Andrew Frados

Writers Club Press
San Jose   New York   Lincoln   Shanghai

Calculations and Constants for Clinical Practice

Writers Club Press
an imprint of iUniverse, Inc.

For information address:
iUniverse, Inc.
5220 S. 16th St., Suite 200
Lincoln, NE 68512
www.iuniverse.com

ISBN: 0-595-21503-3

Printed in the United States of America

To my Wife, JoAnn, for her support,
dedication and love.

CONTENTS

ABBREVIATIONS

A

A–Absorbance; Adenosine; Alveolar Gas; Ampere; Accommodation

a–Absorption; Acidity; Area; Arterial; Asymmetric; Apical

A1–Aortic Component of First Heart Sound

A2–Aortic Component of Second Heart Sound

AA–Achievement Age; Alcoholics Anonymous; Amino Acid; Aminoacyl

AAA–Abdominal Aortic Aneurysm; American Academy of Allergy; American Association of Anatomists

AAAA–American Academy of Anesthesiologist's Assistants

AAAHE–American Association for the Advancement of Health Education

AAAS–American Association for the Advancement of Science

AAB–American Association of Bioanalysts

AABB–American Association of Blood Banks

AAC–Antibiotic-Associated Pseudomembranous Colitis

AACCN–American Association of Critical Care Nurses

AACIA–American Association for Clinical Immunology and Allergy

AACP–American Academy of Cerebral Palsy; American Academy of Child Psychiatry

AADP–American Academy of Denture Prosthetics

AADR–American Academy of Dental Radiology

AADS–American Academy of Dermatology and Syphilology; American Association of Dental Schools

AAE–American Association of Endodontists

AAEGS–American Electroencephalographic Society

AAFP–American Academy of Family Physicians

AAGP–American Academy of of General Practice; Anerican Association of Geriatric Psychiatry

AAHA–American Academy of Health Administration

AAI–American Association of Immunologists

AAID–American Academy of Implant Dentures (or Dentistry)

AAIN–American Association of Industrial Nurses

AAM–American Academy of Microbiology

AAMA–American Association of Medical Assistants

AAMRL–American Association of Medical Record Librarians

AAN–American Academy of Neurology; American Academy of Nursing

AANA–American Association of Nurse Anesthetists

AANM–American Association of Nurse-Midwives

AAO–American Academy of Ophthalmology; American Academy of
    Optometry; American
Academy of Osteopathy; American Academy of Otolaryngology; American Association of Orthodontists

AAOHN–American Association of Occupational Health Nursing

AAOO–American Academy of Ophthalmology and Otolaryngology

AAOP–American Academy of Oral Pathology; American Academy of
    Orthodontists and Prosthetists

AAOS–American Academy of Orthopedic Surgeons

AAP–American Academy of Pediatrics; American Academy of
    Pedodontics; American Academy of Periodontology; American
    Association of Pathologists; Association for the Advancement of
    Psychotherapy; Association of American Physicians

AAPA–American Academy of Physician Assistants

AAPMR–American Academy of Physical Medicine and Rehabilitation

AAPS–American Association of Plastic Surgeons; American Association
    of Physicians and Surgeons

AART–American Association for Respiratory Therapy

AAS–Aortic Arch Syndrome

AAT–Alanine Aminotransferase

AAVV–Accumulated Alveolar Ventilatory Volume

Ab–Antibody; Abnormal

ABC–Aspiration,Biopsy,Cytology; Adriamycin, BCNU, Cyclophos-
   phamide; Airway, Breathing, Circulation; Apnea, Bradycardia,
   Cyanosis; Alternate Birthing Center; Absolute Band Count; Absolute
   Basophil Count

ABCM–Adriamycin,Bleomycin,Cyclophosphamide and Mitomycin C

ABCP–American Board of Cardiovascular Perfusion

ABD–Adriamycin,Bleomycin,DTIC; Abdomen; Abduction

ABDIC–Adriamycin,Bleomycin,DIC,CCNU,Prednisone

ABDV–Adriamycin,Bleomycin,DTIC,Vinblastine

ABE–Antitoxin Botulism Equine; Acute Bacterial Endocarditis

ABG–Arterial Blood Gas

Abl–Abelson Murine Leukemia Virus

ABLB–Alternate Biaural Loudness Balance

ABMS–Advisory Board for Medical Specialties

ABMT–Autologous Bone Marrow Transplantation

ABNM–American Board of Nuclear Medicine

ABP–Adriamycin,Bleomycin,Prednisone

ABPA–Allergic Bronchopulmonary Aspergillosis

ABPP–Bleopirimine

ABR–Absolute Bed Rest; Auditory Brain Response; Agglutination Test
   for Brucellosis

ABS FEB–Absente febre (without fever)

ABV–Adriamycin,Bleomycin,Vinblastine; Actinomycin D, Bleomycin,
   Vincristine

ABVD–Adriamycin,Bleomycin,Vinblastine,Decarbazine

AC–Acromioclavicular; Anodal Closure; Aortic Closure; Axiocervical;
   Anodal Closure; Air Conduction; Adriamycin,CCNU; Acetyl;
   Before Meals; Acetyl; Arabinosylcytosine Abdominal Circumference

Ac–Actinium (Chemical Symbol)

ACA–Acyclovir; Adenocarcinoma; American Chiropractic Association;
   Anterior Cerebral Artery

ACB–Alveolar-Capillary Block; Aortocoronary Bypass

ACBE–Air-Contrast Barium Enema

ACBG–Aortocoronary Bypass Graft

ACC–Accomodation; Acinic Cell Carcinoma; Adenoid Cystic Carcinoma; Adrenocortical Carcinoma; Acute Care Center; Anodal Closure Contraction; Ambulatory Care Center

ACCL–Anodal Closure Clonus

ACD–Acid-Citrate-Dextrose Solution; Absolute Cardiac Dullness; Allergic Contact Dermatitis; Anterior Chamber Diameter; Anterior Chest Diameter; Area of Cardiac Dullness

ACE–Adrenal Cortical Extract; Adriamycin, Cyclophosphamide, Etoposide; Alcohol, Chloroform,Ether; Angiotensin-Converting Enzyme

ACEI–Angiotensin-Converting Enzyme Inhibitor

AcG–Accelerator Globulin (Coagulation Factor V)

ACH–Acetylcholine; Adrenal Cortical Hormone; Arm,Chest,Height

ACI–Acoustic Comfort Index; Adrenal Cortical Insufficiency; Anticlonus Index

ACID–Adriamycin,Cyclophosphamide,Dacarbazine and Actinomycin D

ACIP–Advisory Committee on Immunization Practices

ACL–Acromioclavicular Line; Anterior Cruciate Ligament

ACLA–American Clinical Laboratory Association

ACLPS–Academy of Clinical Laboratory Physicians and Scientists

ACLS–Advanced Cardiac Life Support

ACM–Adriamycin,Cyclophosphamide and Methotrexate; Albumin-Calcium-Magnesium

ACOP–Adriamycin,Cyclophosphamide,Oncovin,Prednisone

ACP–Acyl Carrier Protein; Aspirin,Caffeine,Phenacetin; Anodal Closing Picture; Acid Phosphatase; Association of Clinical Pathologists

ACPS–Acrocephalosyndactyly

ACR–Acriflavine; Anticonstipation Regimen

ACS–American Cancer Society; American Chemical Society; Anodal Closing Sound; Antireticular Cytotoxic Serum; Arterial Cannulation Support

ACTH–Adrenocorticotropic Hormone

AD–Admitting Diagnosis; Adenovirus; Alzheimer's Disease; Analgesic dose; Anodal Duration; Axis Deviation; Axiodistal; Autonomic Dysreflexia; auris dextra (right ear)

ADA–American Dental Association; American Diabetes Association; American Dietetic Association; American Dermatological Association; Anterior Descending Artery

ADAA–American Dental Assistants Association

ADBC–Adriamycin,DTIC,Bleomycin,CCNU

ADC–AIDS Dementia Complex

ADCC–Antibody-Dependent Cell-Mediated Cytotoxicity

ADCONFU–Adriamycin,Cyclophosphamide,5-Fluorouracil and Actinomycin D

ADD–Adduction; Androstanediene; Attention Deficit Disorder; Average Daily Dose

DDS–American Digestive Disease Society

ADE–Acute Disseminated Encephalitis; Apparent Digestible Energy

Ade–Adenine

ADEM–Acute Disseminated Encephalomyelitis

ADH–Alcohol Dehydrogenase; Antidiuretic Hormone

ADHA–American Dental Hygienists' Association

ADHIB–adhibendus (to be administered)

ADI–American Documentation Institute; Acceptable Daily Intake; Axiodistoincisal

ADIC–Adriamycin and Decarbazine

ADL–Activities of Daily Living

ADM–Adriamycin; abductor digiti minimi

AdM–Adrenal Medulla

ADMOV–Admove (apply)

ADMS–Assistant Director of Medical Services

adn–Adenoid

ADO–Axiodisto-occlusal

ADOAP–Adriamycin,Oncovin,ara-C,Prednisone

ADODM–Adult-Onset Diabetes Mellitus

ADOP–Adriamycin,Oncovin,Prednisone

ADP–Academy of Dental Prosthetics; Adenosine Diphosphate; Area Diastolic Pressure

ADPL–Average Daily Patient Load

ADQ–abductor digiti quinti

ADR–Accepted Dental Remedies; Adverse Drug Reaction; Adrenalin; Adriamycin

ADS–American Denture Society; Anatomical Dead Space; Anonymous Donor's Sperm; Antibody Deficiency Syndrome; Antidiuretic Substance

ADT–Adenosine Triphosphate; Alternate-Day Treatment; Agar-Gel Diffusion Test; Accepted Dental Therapeutics

ADV–Adenovirus

ADX–Adrenalectomized

AE–Above-Elbow; Acrodermatitis Enteropathica; Air Entry; Anoxic Encephalopathy

AEA–Above-Elbow Amputation

AED–Automated External Defibrillator

AEG–Air Encephalogram

AEI–Acrylic Eye Illustrator

AEM–Analytical Electron Microscopy

AEP–Artificial Endocrine Pancreas; Auditory Evoked Potential; Average Evoked Potential

AER–Acoustic Evoked Response; Aldosterone Excretion Rate; Auditory Evoked Response; Average Evoked Response

AES–American Encephalographic Society; American Endocrine Society; Antiembolic Stockings; Antral Ethmoidal Sphenoidectomy

AESP–Applied Extrasensory Projection

AET–Absorption Equivalent Thickness

AF–Abnormal Frequency; Albumose-free; Amniotic Fluid; Anterior Fontanelle; Antibody-Forming; Aortic Flow; Atrial Fibrillation; Atrial Flutter; Auricular Fibrillation; Audio-frequency

AFB–Acid-Fast Bacillus; Aflatoxin B; Aortofemoral Bypass

AFBG–Aortofemoral Bypass Graft

AFC–Antibody-Forming Cell

AFG–Aflatoxin G; Alpha Fetal Globulin; Amniotic Fluid Glucose

AFH–Anterior Facial Height

AFI–Amaurotic Familial Idiocy

AFL–Aflatoxicol; Antifatty Liver; Atrial Flutter

AFM–Aflatoxin M

AFO–Ankle-Foot Orthosis

AFP–Alpha-Fetoprotein; Atrial Filling Pressure; Anterior Faucial Pillar

AFPP–Acute Fibrinopurulent Pneumonia

AFQ–Aflatoxin Q

AFR–Aqueous Flare Response

AFRD–Acute Febrile Respiratory Disease

AFS–Acid-Fast Smear; American Fertility Society

AFSP–Acute Fibrinoserous Pneumonia

AFT–Aflatoxin

AFTC–Apparent Free Testosterone Concentration

AFTN–Autonomously Functioning Thyroid Nodule

AFV–Amniotic Fluid Volume

AG–Albumin-Globulin; Aminoglcoside; Anion Gap; Antiglobulin; Atrial Gallop; Axiogingival

Ag–Antigen; Silver (Chemical Symbol)

AGA–Accelerated Growth Area; Acute Gonococcal Arthritis; American Gastroenterological Association; American Geriatrics Association; American Goiter Association; Appropriate forGestational Age; At Gestational Age; Average for Gestational Age; N-acetylglutamate

AGC–Absolute Granulocyte Count; Automatic Gain Control

AGD–Agar-Gel Diffusion; Agarose Diffusion

AGE–Acrylamide Gel Electrophoresis; Acute Gastroenteritis; Agarose Gel Electrophoresis; Angle of Greatest Extension

AGF–Angle of Greatest Flexion

AGG–Agammaglobulinemia; Agammaglobulinemia Leukemia

AGGS–Antigas Gangrene Serum

AGH–Antihemophilic Globulin (Factor VIII)

AGL–Acute Granulocytic Leukemia; Aminoglutethemide

AGN–Acute Glomerulonephritis; Agnosia

AGOS–American Gynecological and Obstetrical Society

AGP–Acid Glycoprotein; Agar-Gel Precipitation

AGPA–American Group Practice Association; American Group Psychotherapy Association

AGR–Anticipatory Goal Response

AGS–Adrenogenital Syndrome; American Gynecological Society

AGT–Antiglobulin Test

AGTH–Adrenoglomerulotropin Hormone

AGTT–Abnormal Glucose Tolerance Test

AGV–Aniline Gentian Violet

AH–Abdominal Hysterectomy; Acetohexamide; Amenorrhea and Hirsutism; Aminohippurate; Antihyaluronidase; Arterial Hypertension; Artificial Heart; Ascites Hepatoma; Autonomic Hyperreflexia

AHA–Acetohydroxamic Acid; Acquired Hemolytic Anemia; American Heart Association; American Hospital Association; Anterior Hypothalamic Area; Autoimmune Hemolytic Anemia; Australian Hepatitis Antigen

AHC–Acute Hemorrhagic Conjunctivitis; Acute Hemorrhagic Cystitis

AHD–Arteriosclerotic Heart Disease; Autoimmune Hemolytic Disease

AHDP–Azacycloheptane-diphosphate

AHE–Acute Hemorrhagic Encephalomyelitis

AHF–Acute Heart Failure; American Health Foundation; American Hepatic Foundation; American Hospital Formulary; Antihemolytic Factor (VIII); Associated Health Foundation

AHG–Aggregated Human Globulin; Antihemophilic Globulin (VIII); Antihuman Globulin

AHGS–Acute Herpetic Gingival Stomatitis

AHLE–Acute Hemorrhagic Leukoencephalitis

AHLS–Antihuman Lymphocyte Serum

AHP–Acute Hemorrhagic Pancreatitis; American Health Professionals

AHS–American Hospital Society; American Hearing Society

AHT–Antihyaluronidase Titer; Augmented Histamine Test; Autoantibodies to Human Thyroglobulin

AHTG–Antihuman Thymocytic Globulin

AHTP–Antihuman Thymocytic Plasma

AI–Accidental Injury; Allergy Index; Angiogenesis Inhibitor; Angiotensin I; Anxiety Index; Aortic Incompetence; Aortic Insufficiency; Apical Impulse; Artificial Insemination; Atherogenic Index; Axioincisal

AIA–Acquired Artery Immune Augmentation; Allylisopropylacetamide; Amylase-Inhibitor Activity

AI-Ab–Anti-Insulin Antibody

AICA–Anterior Inferior Cerebellar Artery; Anterior Internal Cerebral Artery; Anterior Inferior Communicating Artery

AICD–Automatic Implantable Cardiac Defibrillator

AICF–Autoimmune Complement Fixation

AID–Acquired Immunodeficiency Disease; Acute Infectious Disease; Anti-Inflammatory Drug; Artificial Insemination by Donor; Autoimmune Disease

AIE–Acute Inclusion Body Encephalitis

AIEP–Amount of Insulin Extractable from the Pancreas

AIF–Anti-Invasion Factor; Aortoiliofemoral

AIGA–Absence of Immunoglobulin A

AIGM–Absence of Immunoglobulin M

AIH–American Institute of Homeopathy; Artificial Insemination by Husband

AIHA–Autoimmune Hemolytic Anemia

AIL–Angioimmunoblastic Lymphadenopathy

AILD–Angioimmunoblastic Lymphadenopathy with Dysproteinemia

AIle–Alloisoleucine

AIM–Amputees in Motion; L-asparaginase,Ifosfamide and Methotrexate

AIMS–Abnormal Involuntary Movement Scale

AIN–Acute Interstitial Nephritis; American Institute of Nutrition

AINS–Anti-Inflammatory Nonsteroidal

AIO–Amyloid of Immunoglobulin Origin

AION–Anterior Ischemic Optic Neuropathy

AIP–Acute Intermittent Prophyria; Aldosterone-Induced Protein; Anatuberculin,Petragnani's Integral; Automated Immunoprecipitation; Average Intravascular Pressure

AIPS–American Institute of Pathological Science

AIR–Accelerated Idioventricular Rhythm

AIS–Androgen Insensitivity Syndrome; Anti-Insulin Serum

AITT–Arginine Insulin Tolerance Test

AIU–Absolute Iodine Uptake

AIUM–American Institute of Ultrasound in Medicine

AIVR–Accelerated Idioventricular Rhythm

AJ–Ankle Jerk

AJCCS–American Joint Committee on Cancer Staging

AK–Above-Knee; Actinic Keratosis

AKA–Above-Knee Amputation; Alcoholic Ketoacidosis; All Known Allergies

AL–Acute Leukemia; Albumin; Alignment Mark; Axiolingual

Al–Aluminum (Chemical Symbol)

ALA–American Laryngological Association; American Lung Association; Aminolevulinic Acid; Axiolabial

Ala–Alanine

ALAD–Abnormal Left Axis Deviation

ALAG–Axiolabiogingival

ALAT–Alanine Aminotransferase

ALC–Acute Lethal Catatonia; Approximate Lethal Concentration; Axiolinguocervical

ALD–Adrenoleukodystrophy; Alcoholic Liver Disease; Aldolase

ALEP–Atypical Lymphoepitheloid Cell Proliferation

ALF–American Liver Foundation

ALFT–Abnormal Liver Function Tests

ALG–Antilymphocyte Globulin; Axiolinguogingival

ALH–Anterior Lobe Hormone; Anterior Lobe of Hypophysis

ALKAPT–Homogentistic Acid

ALL–Acute Lymphatic Leukemia; Acute Lymphoblastic Leukemia; Acute Lymphocytic Leukemia

ALLO–Atypical Legionella-Like Organisms

ALM–Acral Lentiginous Melanoma; Alveolar Lining Material

ALMI–Anterolateral Myocardial Infarction

ALN–Anterior Lymph Node

ALO–Axiolinguo-occlusal

ALOMAD–Adriamucin,Chlorambucil,Vincristine,Methotrexate,Actin omycin D and Dacarbazine

ALOS–Average Length of Stay

ALP–Alkaline Phosphatase; Anterior Lobe of the Pituitary; Antilymphocyte Plasma

ALRI–Anterolateral Rotational Instability

ALROS–American Laryngological,Rhinological and Otological Society

ALS–Acute Lateral Sclerosis; Amyotrophic Lateral Sclerosis; Angiotensin-Like Substance; Anterolateral Sclerosis; Antilymphocyte Serum; Antilymphatic Serum

ALT–Alanine Aminotransferase; Argon Laser Trabeculoplasty

ALTB–Acute Laryngotracheobronchitis

Alvx–Alveolectomy

ALWMI–Anterolateral Wall Myocardial Infarction

A-Lym–Atypical Lymphocyte

AM–Actomyosin; Alveolar Macrophage; Amalgam; Ampicillin; Amplitude Modulation; Anovular Menstruation; Anteromeatal; Arousal Mechanism; Arterial mean; Atrial Myxoma; Axiomesial; Myopic Astigmatism

Am–Americium (Chemical Symbol)

AMA–Against Medical Advice; American Medical Association

AMB–Amphotericin B

AMBL–Acute Myeloblastic Leukemia

AMC–Antimalaria Campaign; Arm Muscle Circumference; Arthrogryposis Multiplex Congenita; Axiomesiocervical

AMD–Age-Related Macular Degeneration; Alpha-Methyldopa; Axiomesiodistal

AMEA–American Medical Encephalographic Association

AMegL–Acute Megakaryoblastic Leukemia

AMG–Acoustic Myography; Antimacrophage Globulin; Axiomesiogingival

Amh–Mixed Astigmatism with Myopia Predominating

AMI–Acute Myocardial Infarction; Amitryptyline Hydrochloride; Anterior Myocardial Infarction; Association of Medical Illustrators; Axiomesioincisal

AML–Acute Monocytic Leukemia; Acute Myeloblastic Leukemia; Acute Myelocytic Leukemia;

Acute Myelogenous Leukemia; Acute Myeloid Leukemia; Anterior Mitral Leaflet

AMLR–Autologous Mixed Lymphocyte Reaction

AMLS–Antimouse Lymphocyte Serum

AMM–Agnogenic Myeloid Metaplasia; Antibodies to Murine Cardiac Myosin

AMML–Acute Monomyelocytic Leukemia; Acute Myelomonoblastic Leukemia

AMMOL–Acute Myelomonoblastic Leukemia

AMO-Axiomesio-occlusal

AMOL–Acute Monoblastic Leukemia; Acute Monocytic Leukemia

AMP–Acid Mucopolysaccharide; Adenosine Monophosphate; Amphetamine; Average Mean Pressure; Amputation

AMPA–American Medical Publishers Association

AMPPPE–Acute Multifocal Posterior Placoid Pigment Epitheliopathy

AMPS–Abnormal Mucopolysacchariduria; Acid Mucopolysaccharides

AMPT–Aminopterin

AMR–Activity Metabolic Rate; Alternating Motion Rate; Alternating Motion Reflexes; Alternating Motor Rates

AMRI–Anteromedial Rotational Instability

AMS–Acute Mountain Sickness; Antimacrophage Serum; Atypical Measles Syndrome; Auditory Memory Span; Automated Multiphasic Screening

AMSA–Acridinylamine Methanesulphalon-m-anisidide; Amsacrine

AmSECT–American Society of Extra-Corporeal Technology

AMSIT–Appearance,Mood,Sensorium,Intelligence and Thought Processes

AMT–Alpha-Methyltyrosine; American Medical Technologists; Amethpterin; Amphetamine

amu–Atomic Mass Unit

AMV–Assisted Mechanical Ventilation

AMY–Amylase

AN–Anesthesia; Aneurysm; Anisometropia; Anodal; Anorexia Nervosa; Antenatal; Aseptic Necrosis

An–Actinon

ANA–American Narcolepsy Association; American Neurological Association; American Nurses' Association; Antinuclear Antibodies

ANAD–Anorexia Nervosa and Associated Disorders

ANA-FL–Antinuclear Antibody Fluid

ANAP–Agglutination Negative, Absorption Positive

ANC–Absolute Neutrophil Count

AnCC–Anodal Closure Contraction

AND–Anterior Nasal Discharge

AnDTe–Anodal Duration Tetanus

ANF–American Nurses' Foundation; Antinuclear Factor; Atrial Natriuretic Factor

ANIS–Anisocytosis

ANL–Acute Nonlymphoblastic Leukemia

ANLL–Acute Nonlymphoblastic Leukemia; Acute Nonlymphocytic Leukemia; Acute Nonlymphoid Leukemia

AnOC–Anodal Opening Contraction

ANP–Adult Nurse Practitioner; Alpha-atrial Natriuretic Polypeptide; A-Norprogesterone

ANRL–Antihypertensive Neutral Renomedullary Lipids

ANS–Anterior Nasal Spine; Antineutrophilic Serum; Arteriolenephrosclerosis; Autonomic Nervous System

ANSI–American National Standards Institute

ANT–Acoustic Noise Test; Animal Naming Test; Anterior

ANTI–Antibody

ANTR–Apparent Net Transfer Rate

ANUG–Acute Necrotizing Ulcerative Gingivitis

AO–Acid Output; Anodal Opening; Anterior Oblique; Aorta; Aortic Opening; Axio-Occlusal; Opening of the Atrioventricular Valves; Acoustic-Optic; Aortic

AOA–Abnormal Oxygen Affinity; American Optometric Association; American Orthopedic Association; American Osteopathic Association

AOAS–American Osteopathic Academy of Sclerotherapy

AOB–Accessory Olfactory Bulb

AOC–Abridged Ocular Chart; American Ophthalmological Color Chart; Anodal Opening Contraction; Area of Concern

AOCI–Anodal Opening Clonus

AOD–Academy of Operative Dentistry; Adult Onset Diabetes; Arterial Occlusive Disease;

Auriculo-osteodysplasia

AODM–Adult Onset Diabetes Mellitus

AOHA–American Osteopathic Hospital Association

AOIVM–Angiographically Occult Intracranial Vascular Malformation

AOL–Acro-osteolysis

AOM–Acute Otitis Media

AOMA–American Occupational Medical Association

AOO–Anodal Opening Odor

AOP–Anodal Opening Picture

AoP–Left ventricle to Aorta Pressure Gradient

AOPA–American Orthotics and Prosthetics Association

AORN–Association of Operating Room Nurses

AOS–American Ophthalmological Society; American Orthodontic Society; American Otological Society; Anodal Opening Sound

AOSD–Adult-Onset Still's Disease

AOSSM–American Orthopedic Society for Sports Medicine

AOT–Association of Occupational Therapists; Antiovotransferrin

AOTA–American Occupational Therapy Association

AOTe–Anodal Opening Tetanus

AOU–Apparent Oxygen Utilization

AP–Abdominoperineal; Acid Phosphatase;Alkaline Phosphatase; Alum-Precipitated; Angina Pectoris; Antepartum;Anteroposterior; Aortic Pressure; Apical Pulse; Appendicitis; Arterial Pressure; Artificial Pneumothorax; Atrium Pace; axiopulpal

APA–Aldosterone-Producing Adenoma; American Pancreatic Association; American Pharmaceutical Association; American Physiotherapy Association; American Podiatry Association; American

Psychiatric Association; American Psychoanalytic Association; American Psychological Association; American Psychopathological Association; American Psychotherapy Association; Antipernicious Anemia

APAF–Antipernicious Anemia Factor

APAS–Annular Phased-Array System

APB–Atrial Premature Beat; abductor pollicis brevis

APC–Acetylsalicyclic Acid,Phenacetin and Caffeine; Acridinylamine Methanesulphon-M-Anisidide,Prednisone and Chlorambucil; Adenoidal, Pharyngeal, Conjunctival; Antiphlogistic Corticoid; Apneustic Center; Atrial Premature Contraction

APC-C–Aspirin,Phenacetin,Caffeine with Codeine

APCD–Adult Polycystic Disease

APCF–Acute Pharyngoconjunctival Fever

APCG–Apex Cardiogram

APD–Action Potential Duration; Afferent Pupillary Defect; Anterior-Posterior Diameter; Atrial Premature Depolarization; Automated Peritoneal Dialysis

APE–Acute Pulmonary Edema; Aminophylline,Phenobarbital and Ephedrine; Anterior Pituitary Extract

APGAR–Adaptability,Partnership,Growth,Affection and Resolve; American pediatric Gross Assessment Record

APGL–Alkaline Phosphatase Activity of the Granular Leukocytes

APH–Antepartum Hemorrhage; Anterior Pituitary Hormone

APhA–American Pharmaceutical Association

APHP–Anti-Pseudomonas Human Plasma

APIC–Association for Practitioners in Infection Control

APKD–Adult Polycystic Kidney Disease

APL–abductor pollicis longus; Accelerated Painless Labor; Acute Promyelocytic Leukemia; Anterior Pituitary-Like

APM–Academy of Parapsychology and Medicine; Academy of Physical Medicine; Anterior Papillary Muscle

APMR–Association for Physical and Mental Rehabilitation

APN–Acute Pyelonephritis

APO–Adriamycin,Prednisone, and Oncovin; Apomorphine

apo E–Apolipoprotein E

App–Appendix

APPA–American Psychopathological Association

APPG–Aqueous Procaine Penicillin G

APPR–Approaching Lactate Dehydrogenase (1:2 Flip)

APR–Abdominoperineal Resection; Anterior Pituitary Resection; Anatomic Porous Replacement

APRO–Apobarbital

AProL–Acute Progranulocytic Leukemia; Acute Promyelocytic Leukemia

APS–Adenine Phosphosulfate; American Pediatric Society; American Psychological Society; American Proctological Society; American Prosthodontic Society; American Psychological Society; American Psychosomatic Society

APSAC–Anisoylated Plasminogen Streptokinase Activator Complex

APT–Alum-Precipitated Toxoid

APTA–American Physical therapy Association

APTT–Activated Partial Thromboplastin Time

APUD–Amine Precursor Uptake and Decarboxylation

APVD–Anomalous Pulmonary Venous Drainage

APVT–Ammons Picture Vocabulary Test

AQ–Accomplishment Quotient; Achievement Quotient

AR–Achievement Ratio; Active Resistance; Allergic Rhinitis; Androgen Receptor; Aortic Regurgitation; Apical-Radial; Argyll Robertson (Pupil); Arsphenamine; Articulare; Artificial Respiration; Artificially Ruptured; Autoradiography

Ar–Argon (Chemical Symbol)

ARA–Academy of Rehabilitative Audiometry; American Rheumatism Association

ARA-A–Adenine Arabinose

ARA-C–Cytosine Arabinose

ARAS–Ascending Reticular Activating System

ARBOR–Arthropod-borne

ARC–Accelerating Rate Calorimeter; Acquired Immunodeficiency Syndrome Related Complex; Addiction Research Center; American red Cross; Anomalous Retinal Correspondence; Arcuate Nucleus; Arthritis Rehabilitation Center; Association for Retarded Children

ARCA–Acquired Red Cell Aplasia

ARD–Acute Respiratory Disease; Adult Respiratory Distress; Anorectal Dressing; Antibiotic Removal Device; Arthritis and Rheumatic Diseases

ARDS–Adult Respiratory Distress Syndrome

ARF–Acute Renal Failure; Acute Rheumatic Fever; Addiction Research Foundation

Arg–Arginine

ARI–Airway Reactivity Index

ARLD–Alcohol-Related Liver Disease

ARM–Allergy Relief Medicine; Alternating Rate of Motion; Artificial Rupture of Membranes

ARN–Association of Rehabilitation Nurses

ARNP–Advanced Registered Nurse Practitioner

AROM–Active Range of Motion; Artificial Rupture of Membranes

ARP–American Registry of Pathologists

ARPT–American Registry of Physical Therapists

ARRS–American Roentgen Ray Society

ARRT–American Registered Respiratory Therapist; American Registry of Radiologic Technologists

ARS–Adult Recovery Services; American Radium Society; American Rhinologic Society; Antirabies Serum

Ars–Arsphenamine

ARSA–American Reye's Syndrome Association

ARSM–Acute Respiratory System Malfunction

ART–Absolute Retention Time; Accredited Record Technician; Achilles Tendon Reflex Test; Acoustic Reflex Test

ARV–Acquired Immunodefiency Syndrome Associated Retrovirus; Anterior Right Ventricle

AS–Acetylstrophanthidin; Active Sleep; Adams-Stokes; Alveolar Sac; Anal Sphincter; Ankylosing Spondylitis; Antiserum; Aortic Sac; Aortic Stenosis; Aqueous Solution; Atherosclerosis; Audiogenic Seizure; auris sinistra (left ear)

ASA–Acetylsalicylic Acid; American Society of Anesthesiologists; American Standards Association; American Stomatological Association

ASAA–Acquired Severe Aplastic Anemia

ASAHP–American Society of Allied Health Professions

ASAIO–American Society for Artificial Internal Organs

ASAP–As Soon as Possible

ASB–American Society of Bacteriologists

ASBS–Arteriosclerotic Brain Syndrome

ASC–Altered State of Consciousness; Ambulatory Surgery Center; American Society of Cytology; Anterior Subcapsular Cataract; Ascorbic Acid

ASCAD–Arteriosclerotic Coronary Artery Disease

ASCH–American Society of Clinical Hypnosis

ASCLT–American Society of Clinical Laboratory Technicians

ASCMS–American Society of Contemporary Medicine and Surgery

ASCO–American Society of Clinical Oncology; American Society of Contemporary Ophthal-mology

ASCP–American Society of Clinical Pathologists

ASCR–American Society of Chiropodical Roentgenology

ASCVD–Arteriosclerotic Cardiovascular Disease

ASCVRD–Arteriosclerotic Cardiovascular Renal Disease

ASD–Aldosterone Secretion Defect; Atrial Septal Defect

ASDA–American Society of Dental Aesthetics

ASDC–American Society of Dentistry for Children; Association of Sleep Disorders Centers

ASDH–Acute Subdural Hematoma

ASDR–American Society of Dental Radiographers

ASE–Acute Stress Erosion; American Society of Echocardiography; Axilla,Shoulder,Elbow

ASECT–American Society of Extra-Corporeal Technology

ASET–American Society of Electroencephalographic Technologists

ASF–Aniline,Formaldehyde and Sulfur

ASG–American Society for Genetics

ASGD–American Society of Geriatric Dentistry

ASGE–American Society of Gastrointestinal Endoscopy

ASH–American Society for Hematology; Asymmetrical Septal Hypertrophy

ASHA–American School Health Association; American Speech and Hearing Association

ASHG–American Society for Human Genetics

ASHI–Association for the Study of Human Infertility

ASHN–Acute Sclerosing Hyaline Necrosis

ASHNS–American Society for Head and Neck Surgery

ASHP–American Society of Hospital Pharmacists

ASIM–American Society of Internal Medicine

ASIS–Anterior Superior Iliac Spine

ASK–Antistreptokinase

ASLO–Antistreptolysin-O

AsM–Myopic Astigmatism

ASMI–Anteroseptal Myocardial Infarction

ASMT–American Society for Medical Technology

ASN–American Society of Nephrology; American Society for Neurochemistry

Asn–Asparagine

ASO–American Society of Orthodontics; Antistreptolysin-O Titer; Arteriosclerosis Obliterans

ASOS–American Society of Oral Surgeons

ASP–Acute Suppurative Parotitis; American Society of Periodontists; American Society of Parasitologists; Area Systolic Pressure

Asp–Aspartic Acid

ASPA–American Society of Podiatric Assistants

ASPM–American Society of Paramedics

ASPO–American Society for Psychoprophylaxis in Obstetrics

ASPRS–Association of Plastic and Reconstructive Surgeons

ASPVD–Arteriosclerotic Peripheral Vascular Disease

ASR–Aldosterone Secretion Rate

ASRT–American Society of Radiologic Technologists

ASS–Anterior Superior Spine

ASSR–Adult Situation Stress Reaction

AST–Angiotensin Sensitivity Test; Aspartate Aminotransferase; Association of Surgical Technologists; Astemizole; Astigmatism

ASTA–Anti-Alpha-Staphylolysin

ASTI–Antispasticity Index

ASTMH–American Society of Tropical Medicine and Hygiene

ASTO–Antistreptolysin-O

ASTZ–Antistreptozyme

ASU–Acute Stroke Unit

ASUTS–American Society of Ultrasound Technical Specialists

ASV–Anodic Stripping Voltammetry; Antisnake Venom; Arterio-Superficial Venous

AT–Achievement Test; Achilles Tendon; Adjunctive Therapy; Aminotransferase; Amitri-ptyline; Anaphylatoxin; Antithrombin; Antitrypsin; Applanation Tonometry; Ataxia-Telangiectasia; Attenuated; Atraumatic

At–Astatine; Atrial

ATA–Alimentary Toxic Aleukia; American Thyroid Association; American Tinnitus Association; Antithyroglobulin Antibody; Anti-Toxoplasma Antibodies

ATB–Antibiotic

ATC–Activated Thymus Cells; Around the Clock

ATD–Alzheimer-Type Dementia; Antithyroid Drug; Asphyxiating Thoracic Dystrophy; Autoimmune Thyroid Disease

ATDC–Association of Thalidomide Damaged Children

ATG–Adenine,Thymine,Guanine; Antihuman Thymocyte Globulin; Antithyroglobulin

ATGAM–Antithymocyte Gamma-Globulin

ATH–Acetylthyrosine Hydrazide

ATHR–Angina Threshold Heart Rate

AT III–Antithrombin III

ATL–Achilles Tendon Lengthening; Adult T-Cell Leukemia; Atypical Lymphocytes

ATLA–Adult T-Cell Leukemia Antigen

ATLS–Advanced Trauma Life Support

ATLV–Adult T-Cell Leukemia Virus

ATN–Acute Tubular Necrosis

ATNC–Atraumatic/Normocephalic

ATNR–Asymmetrical Tonic Neck Reflex

ATP–Adenosine Triphosphate

ATPD–Ambient Temperature and Pressure,Dry

ATPS–Ambient Temperature and Pressure, Saturated with Water Vapor

ATR–Achilles Tendon Reflex; Atrial

ATS–Adjustable Thigh Antiembolism Stockings; American Therapeutic Society; American Thoracic Society; American Trauma Society; Antitetanic Serum; Antithymocyte Serum; Anxiety Tension State; Arteriosclerosis

ATT–Arginine Tolerance Test

ATZ–Atypical Transformation Zone

AU–Allergenic Units; Antitoxin Unit; aures unitas (both ears); Arbitrary Units

Au–Gold (Chemical symbol)

AUA–American Urological Association

AuAg–Australian antigen

AUHAA–Australia Hepatitis-Associated Antigen

AUL–Acute Undifferentiated Leukemia

AUO–Amyloid of Unknown Origin

AUSPE–Audiology and Speech Pathology

AV–Adriamycin and Vincristine; Alveolar Duct; Anterior-Ventral; Anteversion; Aortic Valve; Arteriovenous; Atrioventricular; Auriculoventricular; Avoirdupois

AVA–American Vocational Association; Arteriovenous Anastomosis

AVAF–Anteverted,Anteflexed

AVC–Allantoin Vaginal Cream; Association of Vitamin Chemists; Associative Visual Cortex; Atrioventricular Canal

AVCD–Atrioventricular Canal Defect

AVCS–Atrioventricular Conduction System

AVD–Aortic Valve Disease; Apparent Volume of Distribution

AVE–Aortic Valve Echocardiogram

AVF–Antiviral Factor; Arteriovenous Fistula

AVH–Acute Viral Hepatitis

AVHB–Atrioventricular Heart Block

AVI–Air Velocity Index

AVM–Adriamycin, Vinblastine and Methotrexate; Adriamycin, Vincristine and Mitomycin-C; Arteriovenous Malformation

AVN–Acute Vasomotor Nephropathy; Arteriovenous Nicking; Atrioventricular Node; Avascular Necrosis

AVP–Adriamycin,Vincristine and Procarbazine; Antiviral Protein

AVR–Aortic Valve Replacement

AVRP–Atrioventricular Refractory Period

AVS–Arteriovenous Shunt; Association for Voluntary Sterilization

AVSC–Aortic Valve Cusp Separation

AVSS–Afebrile, Vital Signs Stable

AVT–Allen Vision Test; Area Ventralis of Tsai; Arginine Vasotocin; Atypical Ventricular Tachycardia

AW–Above Waist; Anterior Wall

AWF–Adrenal Weight Factor

AWI–Anterior Wall Infarction

AWMI–Anterior Wall Myocardial Infarction

AWP–Airway Pressure

Ax–Axillary

AXT–Alternating Exotropia

AZ–Aschheim-Zondek

AZA–Azathioprine

AZQ–Aziridinylbenzoquinone; Diaziquone

AZT-Zidovudine

AZU–6-Azauracil

B

B–Bacillus; Bacterium; Balantidium; Bicuspid; Bilateral; Blood; Bordetella; Buccal; Bursa Cells; Body

B–Boron (Chemical symbol)

BA–Backache; Bacterial Agglutination; Basion; Betamethasone Acetate; Bile Acid; Bone Age; Bovine Albumin; Brachial Artery; Breathing Apparatus; Bronchial Asthma; Buccoaxial

Ba–Barium (Chemical Symbol)

BAC–Bacteria; Bacterial Antigen Complex; Benzalkonium Chloride; Bronchoalveolar Cells; Buccoaxiocervical

BACO–Bleomycin, Adriamycin, Lomustine(CCNU) and Vincristine

BACON–Bleomycin, Adriamycin, Lomustine, Vincristine and Nitrogen Mustard

BACOP–Bleomycin, Adriamycin, Cyclophosphamide, Vincristine and Prednisone

BACT–Bleomycin, Adriamycin, Cytoxan and Tamoxifen

BAD–Bipolar Affective Disorder

BAE–Bronchial Artery Embolization

BaE–Barium Enema

BAEP–Brain Stem Auditory Evoked Potential

BAER–Brain Stem Auditory Evoked Response

BAG–Buccoaxiogingival

BAL–Blood Alcohol Level; Bronchoalveolar Lavage; British Anti-Lewisite

BALB–Binaural Alternate Loudness Balance Test

B-ALL–B-Cell Acute Lymphoblastic Leukemia

BAm–Mean Brachial Artery

BaM–Barium Meal

BAMON–Bleomycin, Adriamycin, Methotrexate, Vincristine and Nitrogen Mustard

BAP–Bleomycin, Adriamycin and Prednisone; Brachial Artery Pressure; Bovine Albumin in Phosphate Buffer

BAS–Benzyl Analogue of Serotonin; Benzyl Antiserotonin

BASH–Body Acceleration Synchronous with the Heartbeat

BAVIP–Bleomycin, Dacarbazine, Vincristine, Adriamycin and Prednisone

BAVP–Balloon Aortic Valvuloplasty

BAW–Bronchoalveolar Wash Fluids

BB–Beta-Blocker; Blood Bank; Blood Buffer Base; Blow Bottle; Blue Bloaters; Both Bones; Bowel or Bladder; Breakthrough Bleeding; Breast Biopsy; Bundle-Branch

BBA–Born Before Arrival

BBB–Blood-Brain Barrier; Bundle-Branch Block

BBBB–Bilateral Bundle-Branch Block

BBD–Benign Breast Disease

BBHB–Bundle-Branch Heart Block

BBM–Banked Breast Milk

BBRS–Burks' Behavior Rating Scale

BBS–Bilateral Breath Sounds; Bombesin

BBT–Basal Body Temperature; Blood Bank Technologist

BB to MM–Belly Button to Medial Malleolus

BC–Bactericidal Concentration; Birth Control; Bone Conduction; Bowman's Capsule; Bronchial Carcinoma; Buccal Cartilage; Buccocervical; Bulbocavernosus; Bulbus Chordae

BCA–Balloon Catheter Angioplasty; Basal Cell Atypia; Brachiocephalic Artery

B-CAVe–Bleomycin, CCNU, Adriamycin and Velban

BCC–Basal Cell Carcinoma; Birth Control Clinics

BCD–Basal Cell Dysplasia; Bleomycin,Cyclophosphamide and Dactinomycin

BCE–Basal Cell Epithelioma

BCF–Basophil Chemotactic Factor

BCFP–Breast Cyst Fluid Protein

BCG–Bacille Calmette-Guerin; Ballistocardiogram; Bicolor Guaiac Test; Bilateral Cystograms

BCH–Basal Cell Hyperplasia

BChD–Bachelor of Dental Surgery

BCIC–Birth Control Investigation Committee

B-CLL–B-Cell Lymphatic Leukemia

BCLS–Basic Cardiac Life Support System

BCM–Birth Control Medication

BCOP–Carmustine,Cyclophosphamide,Vincristine and Prednisone

BCP–Birth Control Pill; Blood Pressure Cuff; Basic Calcium Phosphate

BCR–Bulbocalvernosus Reflex

BCS–Battered Child Syndrome; Blood Cell Separator; Budd-Chiari Syndrome

BCSI–Breast Cancer Screening Indicator

BCUPP–Carmustine,Vinblastine,Procarbazine and Prednisone

BCV–Basal Cell Vigilance

BCVP–Carmustine,Cyclophosphamide,Vincristine and Prednisone

BCVPP–Carmustine,Cyclophosphamide,Vinblastine,Prednisone and Procarbazine

BD–Base Deficit; Batten's Disease; Behavioral Disorder; Belladonna; Below Diaphragm; Best Delay; Bile Duct; Binocular Deprivation; Birth Defect; Black Death; Borderline Dull; Brain Dead; Bronchial Drainage; Buccodistal

BDAE–Boston Diagnostic Aphasia Examination

BDC–Burn-Dressing Change

BDE–Bile Duct Examination; Bile Duct Exploration

BDI–Beck Depression Inventory; Burn Depth Indicator

BDIBS–Boston Diagnostic Inventory of Basic Skills

BDM–Border Detection Method

BDOPA–Bleomycin, Dacarbazine, Vincristine, Prednisone and Adriamycin

BDP–Beclomethasone Diproprionate

BDR–Background Diabetic Retinopathy

BDTVMI–Beery Developmental Test of Visual Motor Integration

BDUR–Bromodeoxyuridine

BE–Bacillary Emulsion; Bacterial Endocarditis; Barium Enema; Base Excess; Below Elbow; Bile Esculin; Bovine Enteritis; Bread Equivalent; Breast Examination; Bronchoesophagology

Be–Beryllium (Chemical Symbol)

BEAM–Brain Electrical Activity Mapping

BEAR–Biological Effects of Atomic Radiation

BEC–Bacterial Endocarditis

BEE–Basal Energy Expenditure

BEI–Butanol-Extractable Iodine

BEP–Brain Evoked Potential

BER–Basic Electrical Rhythm

BERA–Brain Stem Evoked Response Audiometry

BES–Balanced Electrolyte Solution

BETA–Beta-Streptococcus Screen

BETS–Benign Epileptiform Transients of Sleep

BF–Bentonite Flocculation; Black Female; Blastogenic Factor; Blood Flow; Bone Fragment; Buffered; Deny's Tuberculin; Lymphocyte Transforming Factor

BFB–Biological Feedback

BFC–Benign Febrile Convulsion

BFL–Bird-Fancier's Lung

BFP–Biologic False-Positive

BFR–Biological False-Positive Reaction; Blood Flow Rate; Bone Formation Rate

BFT–Bentonite Flocculation Test

BFU-E–Burst-Forming Unit

BG–Bender Gestalt; Bicolor Guaiac; Blood Glucose; Bone Graft; Bordet-Gengou; Brilliant Green; Buccogingival

BGC–Basal-Ganglion Calcification; Blood Group Class

BGD–Blood Group-Degrading Enzymes

BGG–Bovine Gamma-Globulin

BGH–Bovine Growth Hormone

BGLB–Brilliant Green Lactose Broth

BGP–Beta-Glycerophosphatase

BGRS–Blood Glucose Reagent Strips

BGS–Blood Group Substance

BGSA–Blood Granulocyte-Specific Activity

BGTT–Borderline Glucose Tolerance Test

BH–Benzalkonium and Heparin; Brain Hormone; Bundle of His

BHA–Butylated Hydroxyanisole

BHAT–Beta-Blocker Heart Attack Trial

BHBA–Beta-Hydroxybutyric Acid

B-HCG–Beta Human Chorionic Gonadotropin

BHD–Carmustine,Hydroxyurea and Dacarbazine

BHD-V–Carmustine,Hydroxyurea,Dacarbazine and Vincristine

BHI–Biosynthetic Human Insulin; Brain-Heart Infusion

BHI-ac–Brain-Heart Infusion Broth with Acetone

BHIB–Beef Heart Infusion Broth

BHIBA–Beef Heart Infusion Broth Agar

BHIS–Beef Heart Infusion Supplement

BHL–Biological Half-Life

BHN–Bephenium Hydroxynaphthoate

BHP–Basic Health Profile

BHR–Basal Heart Rate

BHS–Beta-Hemolytic Streptococcus

BHT–Beta-Hydroxytheophylline; Breath Hydrogen Test; Butylated Hydroxytoluene

BI–Bacteriological Index; Biological Index; Bodily Injury; Bone Injury; Bowel Impaction; Braille Institute; Burn Index

Bi–Bismuth

BIB–Brought in by

BIC–Biomedical Instrumentation Consultant

BiCNU–Bischloroethylnitrosurea,Carmustine, and Nitrosurea

BID–bis in die (Twice a Day)

BIDLB–Block in the Posteroinferior Division of the Left Branch

BIDS–Bedtime Insulin,Daytime Sulfonylurea

BIH–Benign Intracranial Hypertension; Bilateral Inguinal Herniae

BIKE–Therapeutic Protocol: Prednisone and Vincristine and phase two is Methotrexate Followed by 6-Mercaptopurine and then Cyclophosphamide

BIL–Bilirubin

BILI-C–Conjugated Bilirubin

BIMA–Bilateral Internal Mammary Arteries

BIN–Benign Intradermal Nevus

BIP–Bacterial Intravenous Protein; Biparietal Diameter; Bismuth Iodoform Paraffin

BIR–Backward Internal Rotation; Basic Incidence Rate

BiSP–Between Ischial Spines; Bispinous Diameter; Interspinous Diameter

BiT–Between Great Trochanters

BITU–Benzyl-Thiourea

BIV–Bovine Immunodeficiency-Like Virus

BIW–Twice a Week

BJ–Bence Jones; Biceps Jerk; Bone and Joint

BJE–Bones,Joints and Examination

BJM–Bones,Joints and Muscles

BJP–Bence Jones Protein

Bk–Berkelium

BKA–Below the Knee Amputation

BKO–Below-Knee Orthosis

BL–Bessey-Lowry; Blood; Blood Loss; Bone-Marrow-Derived Lymphocyte; Buccolingual; Burkitt's Lymphoma

BLAC–Bladder Urine

BLAD–Borderline Left Axis Deviation

BLB–Boothby-Lovelace-Bulbulian

BLE–Both Lower Extremities

BLEO–Bleomycin Sulfate

BLESS–Bath,Laxative,Enema,Shampoo and Shower

BLG–Beta-Lactoglobulin

BLL–Brows,Lids and Lashes

BLM–Bimolecular Liquid Membrane; Bleomycin Sulfate

BLN–Bronchial Lymph Nodes

BlP–Blood Pressure

BLS–Basic Life Support; Blood and Lymphatic Systems

BLT–Bilateral Tubal Ligation; Bladder Tumor; Blood-Clot Lysis Time

BLU–Bessey-Lowry Units

BLV–Bovine Leukemia Virus

BM–Bachelor of Medicine; Basal Medium; Basal Metabolism; Basement Membrane; Basilar Membrane; Black Male; Body Mass; Bone Marrow; Bowel Movement; Breast Milk; Buccal Mass; Buccomesial

BMA–Bone Marrow Aspiration

BMC–Bone Marrow Cells

BME–Basal Medium, Eagle's; Brief Maximal Effort

BMG–Benign Monoclonal Gammopathy

BMI–Body Mass Index

BMJ–Bones,Muscles and Joints

BMK–Birthmark

BMMP–Benign Mucous Membrane Pemphigus

BMP–Bone Marrow Pressure; Bone Morphogenic Protein; Carmustine,Methotrexate and Procarbazine

BMPP–Benign Mucous Membrane Pemphigus

BMR–Basal Metabolic Rate

BMS–Bachelor of Medical Science; Biomedical Monitoring System; Bleomycin Sulphate

BMT–Bachelor of Medical Technology; Bilateral Myringotomy Tubes; Bone Marrow Transplant; Buschke Memory Test

BMTU–Bone Marrow Transplant Unit

BN–Brachial Neuritis

BNC–Bladder Neck Contracture

BNL–Breast Needle Location

BNMSE–Brief Neuropsychological Mental Status Examination

BNO–Bladder Neck Obstruction; Bowels Not Open

BNPA–Binasal Pharyngeal Airway

BNR–Bladder Neck Resection; Bladder Neck Retraction

BNS–Benign Nephrosclerosis

BO–Bachelor of Osteopathy; Base Out; Behavior Objective; Bowel Obstruction; Bowels Open; Bucco-Occlusal; Bolton; Body Odor

B&O–Belladonna and Opium

Bo–Bohemium; Magnetic Induction Field

BOA–Born on Arrival; Born out of Asepsis

BOCG–Brudzinski,Oppenheim, Chaddock and Gullaird

BOD–Biochemical Oxygen Demand; Biological Oxygen Demand

BOE–Bilateral Otitis Externa

BOLD–Bleomycin,Vincristine,Lomustine and Dacarbazine

BOM–Bilateral Otitis Media

BOMB–Vincristine,Adriamycin,6-Mercaptopurine and Prednisone

BONENT–Board of Nephrology Examiners for Nursing and Technology

BOO–Bladder Outlet Obstruction

BOP–Bleomycin,Vincristine and Prednisone; Buffalo Orphan Prototype

BOPAM–Bleomycin,Vincristine,Prednisone,Adriamycin,Nitrogen Mustard and Methotrexate

BOR–Bowels Open Regularly

BOT–Base of Tongue

BOW–Bag of Waters

BP–Bachelor of Pharmacy; Back Pressure; Barometric Pressure; Bathroom Privileges; Bedpan; Behavior Pattern; Benzoyl Peroxide; Biotic Potential; Biparietal; Blood Pressure; Bronchopleural; Bronchopulmonary; Buccopulpal; Bypass

BPA–Blood Pressure Assembly; Bovine Plasma Albumin

BPD–Biparietal Diameter; Blood Pressure Decreased; Blood Program Directives; Broncho-pulmonary Dysplasia

BPE–Bacterial Phosphatidylethanolamine

BPF–Bronchopleural Fistula

BPG–Blood Pressure Gauge

BPH–Benign Prostatic Hypertrophy; Bypass Graft; Benign Prostatic Hyperplasia

BPI–Blood Pressure Increased

BPL–Benzylpenicilloyl Polylysine; Beta-Propiolactone
BPLN–Bilateral Pelvic Lymph Nodes
BPLND–Bilateral Pelvic Lymph Node Dissection
BPM–Beats Per Minute; Breaths Per Minute; Brompheniramine Maleate
BPMS–Blood Plasma Measuring System
BPN–Bacitracin,Polymyxin B and Neomycin
BPO–Benzylpenicilloyl
BPP–Bovine Pancreatic Polypeptide
BPR–Blood Pressure Recorder
BPRS–Brief Psychiatric Rate Scale
BPS–Beats Per Second; Behavioral Pharmacological Society; Biophysical Society; Breaths Per Second; Brain Protein Solvent
BPSD–Bronchopulmonary Segmental Drainage
BPV–Benign Paroxysmal Vertigo; Benign Positional Vertigo; Bovine Papilloma Virus
Bq–Becquerel
BR–Bathroom; Bedrest; Bilirubin; Bridge
Br–Bromine (Chemical Symbol); Breech; Bridge; Bronchitis; Brucella
BRAO–Branch Retinal Artery Occlusion
BRAT–Banana,Rice Cereal,Apple Sauce (or Toast, or Tea)
BRB–Blood-Retinal Barrier
BRBC–Bovine Red Blood Cells
BRBNS–Blue Rubber-Bleb Nevus Syndrome
BRBPR–Bright Red Blood Per Rectum
BRCM–Below Right Costal Margin
BrDU–5-Bromodeoxyuridine
Brhp–Bronchophony
BRJ–Brachioradialis Jerk
BrM–Breast Milk
BRP–Bathroom Privileges; Bilirubin Production

BS–Bachelor of Surgery; Before Sleep; Binet-Simon; Bismuth Subsalicylate; Blood Sugar; Bloom Syndrome; Bowel Sounds; Breaking Strength; Breath Sounds; Bureau of Standards

B&S–Bartholin's and Skene's (Glands)

BSA–Biofeedback Society of America; Bismuth Sulfite Agar; Body Surface Area; Bovine Serum Albumin

BSAER–Brain Stem Auditory Evoked Response; Brief, Small, Abundant Potentials

BSB–Body Surface Burned

BSC–Bedside Commode; Biological Stain Commission

B-scan–Brightness Modulation Scan

BSDLB–Block in the Anterosuperior Division of the Left Branch

BSE–Bilateral, Symmetrical and Equal; Breast Self Exam

BSER–Brain Stem Evoked Responses

BSF–Backscatter Factor; Busulfan

BSGA–Beta-Streptococcus Group A

BSI–Bound Serum Iron

BSID–Bayley Scales of Infant Development

BSL–Benign Symmetric Lipomatosis; Blood Sugar Level;

BSN–Bachelor of Science in Nursing; Bowel Sounds Normal

BSO–Bilateral Sagittal Osteotomy; Bilateral Salpingo-Oophorectomy; Bilateral Serous Otitis

BSOM–Bilateral Serous Otitis Media

BSOT–Bachelor of Science in Occupational Therapy

BSP–Bromsulphalein

BSPM–Body Surface Potential Mapping

BSR–Basal Skin Resistance; Blood Sedimentation Rate

BSS–Balanced Salt Solution; Black Silk Suture; Brain Stimulation Reinforcement; Buffered Saline Solution

BST–Blood Serological Test; Brief Stimulus Therapy

BSU–Bartholin's, Skene's and Urethral

BT–Bedtime; Bitemporal; Bituberous; Blacky Test; Bladder Tremor; Bladder Tumor; Bleeding Time; Blood Transfusion; Body Temperature; Brain Tumor; Breast Tumor; Carmustine and Triazinate

BTA–Blood Transfusion Association

BTB–Breakthrough Bleeding; Bromothymol Blue

BTBC–Boehm Test of Basic Concepts

BTEA–Boston Test for Examining Aphasia

BTFS–Breast Tumor Frozen Section

BTL–Bilateral Tubal Ligation

BTMD–Batten-Turner Muscular Dystrophy

BTPS–Body Conditions-Body Temperature, Ambient Pressure, and Saturated with Water Vapor

BTR–Bezold-Type Reflex; Bladder Tumor Recheck

BTS–Blood Transfusion Service

BTSG–Brain Tumor Study Group

BTSH–Beef Thyroid-Stimulating Hormone; Bovine Thyrotropin

BTX–Bungarotoxin

BTZ–Butazolidin

BUDU–Bromodeoxyuridine

BUE–Both Upper Extremities

BUG–Buccal Ganglion

BUI–Brain Uptake Index

BUN–Blood Urea Nitrogen; Bunion

BUO–Bilirubin of Unknown Origin; Bleeding of Unknown Origin; Bruising of Unknown Origin

BUR–Backup Rate

BUS–Bartholin's, Urethral and Skene's Glands

BV–Bacitracin V; Biological Value; Blood Vessel; Blood Volume; Bronchovesicular

BVA–Bioimpedance Venous Analysis

BVAP–Carmustine, Vincristine, Adriamycin and Prednisone

BVD–Carmustine, Vincristine and Dacarbazine

BVDT–Brief Vestibular Disorientation Test
BVE–Binocular Visual Efficiency
BVH–Biventricular Hypertrophy
BVI–Blood Vessel Invasion
BVL–Bilateral Vas Ligation
BVM–Bronchovascular Markings
BVMG–Bender Visual-Motor Gestalt
BVP–Blood Vessel Prosthesis
BVRT–Benton Visual Retention Test
BW–Below Waist; Birth Weight; Bladder Washout; Body Water
BWFI–Bacteriostatic Water for Injection
BWS–Battered Woman Syndrome
BWSV–Black Widow Spider Venom
BX–Biopsy
BZ–Benzodiazepine
BZDZ–Benzodiazepine

C

C–Ascorbic Acid; Carbon (chemical symbol); Centigrade; Celsius; Cervical; Chest; Clonus; Cyanosis; Curie; Cathode; Closure; Speed of Light
CA–Cancer; Carbonic Anhydrase; Carcinoma; Cardiac Arrest; Carotid Artery; Cathode; Cerebral Aqueduct; Cervicoaxial; Chronological Age; Celiac Axis; Cold Agglutinin; Commissural-Association; Coronary Arrest; Coronary Artery; Cortisone Acetate; Cytosine Arabinoside
Ca–Calcium (Chemical Symbol); Cancer; Carcinoma; Cathode
CAA–Constitutional Aplastic Anemia
CAAT–Computer-Assisted Axial Tomography
CAB–Coronary Artery Bypass

CABG–Coronary Artery Bypass Graft

CABOP–Cyclophosphamide, Adriamycin, Bleomycin, Oncovin and Prednisone

CAC–Cardiac-Accelerator Center; Cardiac Arrest Code; Comprehensive Ambulatory Care

CACC–Cathodal Closure Contraction

CACI–Computer Assisted Continuous Infusion

$CaCl_2$–Calcium Chloride

$CaCO_3$–Calcium Carbonate

CACP–Cisplatin

CACX–Cancer of the Cervix

CAD–Computer-Assisted Diagnosis; Coronary Artery Disease; Cytosine Arabinoside and Daunomycin

Cad–Cadaver

CADI–Computer-Assisted Diabetic Instruction

CAD-I–Adriamycin, Cyclophosphamide, and Cisplatin

CADIC–Cyclophosphamide, Adriamycin and Dacarbazine

CADL–Communication Abilities in Daily Living

CADTe–Cathodal Duration Tetanus

CAE–Cellulose Acetate Electrophoresis; Contigent After-effects

CAF–Continuous Atrial Fibrillation; Cooley's Anemia Foundation; Cyclophosphamide, Adriamycin and 5-Fluorouracil; Continuous Atrial Flutter

CAFP–Cyclophosphamide, Adriamycin, 5-Fluorouracil and Prednisone

CAFT–Clinitron Air Fluidized Therapy

CADFVP–Cyclophosphamide, Adriamycin, 5-Fluorouracil, Vincristine and Prednisone

CAG–Chronic Atrophic Gastritis

CAH–Chronic Active Hepatitis; Chronic Aggressive Hepatitis; Congenital Adrenal Hyper-plasia

CAHD–Coronary Artery Heart Disease; Coronary Atherosclerotic Heart Disease

CAHEA–Committee on Allied Health Education and Accreditation

CAI–Computer-Assisted Instruction; Confused Artificial Insemination

CAL–Calculated Average Life; Callus; Calories; Chronic Airflow Limitation; Computer-assisted Learning

CALASP–Cytosine Arabinoside, Vincristine, L-Asparaginase and Prednisone

CALD–Chronic Active Liver Disease

CALGB–Cancer and Leukemia Group B

cALL–Common Null Cell Acute Lymphoblastic Leukemia

CAM–Chorioallantoic Membrane; Contralateral Axillary Metastasis; Cyclophosphamide, Adriamycin, Methotrexate and Folic Acid

CAMB–Cyclophosphamide, Adriamycin, Methotrexate and Bleomycin

CAMELEON–Cytosine Arabinoside, High-dose Methotrexate, Citrovorum Factor and Vincristine

CAMF–Cyclophosphamide, Adriamycin, Methotrexate and Fluorouracil; Cyclophospha-mide, Adriamycin, Methotrexate and Folic Acid

CAMP–Christie, Atkins, Munch-Peterson; Computer-assisted Menu Planning; Cyclophosphamide, Adriamycin, Methotrexate and Procarbazine

CAMU–Cardiac Ambulatory Monitoring Unit; Coronary Arrhythmia Monitoring Unit

CAN–Cord Around Neck

CAO–Chronic Airflow Obstruction; Chronic Airway Obstruction

CAOC–Cathodal Opening Contraction

CAP–Cancer of the Prostate; Capillary Blood; Chloramphenicol; Cholesteric Analysis Profile; Compound Action Potentials; Cyclophosphamide, Adriamycin, and Cisplatin; Cyclophos-phamide, Adriamycin and Prednisone

CAPA–Caffeine, Alcohol, Pepper and Aspirin

CAPD–Chronic Ambulatory Peritoneal Dialysis; Continuous Abdominoperitoneal Dialysis; Continuous Ambulatory Peritoneal Dialysis

CAPPA–Caffeine, Alcohol, Pepper, Peppermint and Aspirin

CAPRI–Cardiopulmonary Research Institute

CAPS–Caffeine, Alcohol, Pepper and Spicy Food

CAR–Cardiac Ambulation Routine; Conditioned Avoidance Response

CARF–Commission on Accreditation of Rehabilitation Facilities

CAS–Cancer Attitude Survey; Cardiac Adjustment Scale; Cardiac Surgery; Carotid Artery Stenosis; Cerebral Arteriosclerosis; Control Adjustment Strap

CASHD–Coronary Arteriosclerotic Heart Disease

CASS–Coronary Artery Surgery Study

CAT–Cataract; Children's Apperception Test; Chloramphenicol Acetyltransferase; Choline Acetyltransferase; Classified Anaphylatoxin; Computerized Axial Tomography; Computer-aided Transcription; Cytosine Arabinoside and Thioguanine; Cytosine Arabinoside, Adria-mycin and 6-Thioguanine

CATCH–Community Actions to Control High Blood Pressure

CAV–Congenital Absence of Vagina; Congenital Adrenal Virilism; Cyclophosphamide, Adriamycin and Vincristine

CAVB–Complete Atrioventricular Block

CAVC–Common Arterioventricular Canal

CAVD–Completion, Arithmetic Problems, Vocabulary and Following Directions

CAVE–CCNU, Adriamycin and Vinblastine

CAVH–Continuous Arteriovenous Hemofiltration

CAVP–Cyclophosphamide, Adriamycin, VM-26 and Prednisone

CAVPM–Cyclophosphamide, Adriamycin, VP-16, Prednisone and Methotrexate

CAWA–Closing Abductory Wedge Osteotomy

CB–Carbenicillin; Catheterized Bladder; Ceased Breathing; Cesarean Birth; Chronic Bronchitis; Contrast Baths; Code Blue

CBA–Chronic Bronchitis and Asthma

CBC–Carbenicillin; Complete Blood Count

CBD–Closed Bladder Drainage; Common Bile Duct

CBDE–Common Bile Duct Exploration

CBF–Capillary Blood Flow; Cerebral Blood Flow; Coronary Blood Flow; Cortical Blood Flow

CBFS–Cerebral Blood Flow Studies

CBFV–Cerebral Blood Flow Velocity

CBG–Capillary Blood Gas; Capillary Blood Glucose; Corticosteroid-binding Globulin; Cortisol-Binding Globulin

CBI–Continuous Bladder Irrigation

CBIP–Center Background Interference Procedure

CBL–Cord Blood Leukocytes

CBMMP–Chronic Benign Mucous Membrane Pemphigus

CBN–Chronic Benign Neutropenia

CBPPA–Cytoxan, Bleomycin, Procarbazine, Prednisone and Adriamycin

CBR–Carotid Bodies Resected; Complete Bed Rest; Crude Birth Rate

CBS–Chronic Brain Syndrome

CBV–Central Blood Volume; Circulating Blood Volume

CBW–Critical Bandwidth

CC–Cardiac Catherization; Cardiac Cycle; Cerebral Commissure; Cerebral Concussion; Chief Complaint; Chondrocalcinosis; Choriocarcinoma; Chronic Complainer; Circulatory Collapse; Classical Conditioning; Clinical Course; Closing Capacity; Compound Cathartic; Coracoclavicular; Cord Compression; Corpora Cardiaca; Corpus Callosum; Costochondral; Craniocaudad; Creatinine Clearance; Cubic Centimeter; Current Complaints

CCA–Chimpanzee Coryza Agent; Circumflex Coronary Artery; Common Carotid Artery

CCAP–Capsule Cartilage Articular Preservation

CCAVV–CCNU, Cyclophosphamide, Adriamycin,, Vincristine and VP-16

CCB–Calcium Channel Blocker

CCBB–Clinical Center Blood Bank

CCBV–Central Circulating Blood Volume

CCC–Cathodal Closure Contraction; Chronic Calculous Cholecystitis; Consecutive Case Conference; County Counseling Center; Continuing Community Care

CCCl-Cathodal Closure Clonus

CCCR–Closed-Chest Cardiac Resuscitation

CCE–Clear Cell Carcinoma; Clubbing, Cyanosis and Edema

CCF–Cardiolipin Complement Fixation; Compound Comminuted Fracture; Congestive Cardiac Failure

CCFE–Cyclophosphamide, Cisplatin, Fluorouracil and Estramustine

CCG–Cholecystogram

CCHD–Cyanotic Congenital Heart Disease

CCHS–Congenital Central Hypoventilation Syndrome

CCI–Chronic Coronary Insufficiency

CCJ–Costochondral Junction

CCK–Cholecystokinin

CCL–Carcinoma Cell Line; Critical Carbohydrate Level

CCM–Cyclophosphamide, CCNU and Methotrexate

CCMA–CCNU, Cyclophosphamide, Methotrexate and Adriamycin

CCMS–Clean-Catch Midstream

CCN–Coronary Care Nursing

CCNS–Cell Cycle Nonspecific

CCNU–Lomustine

CCNU-OP–Lomustine, Oncovin and Prednisone

CCOB–CCNU, Cyclophosphamide, Oncovin and Bleomycin

C-collar–Cervical Collar

CCP–Ciliocytophthoria; Certified Cardiovascular Perfusionist

CCPD–Continuous Cyclical Peritoneal Dialysis

CCPDS–Centralized Cancer Patient Data System

CCR–Continuous Complete Remission

CCRN–Critical Care Registered Nurse

CCS–Cell-Cycle-Specific; Clinical Sleep Society; Concentration Camp Syndrome; Crippled Children's Society

CC&S–Cornea, Conjunctiva and Sclera

CCT–Chocolate-Coated Tablet; Coated Compressed Tablet; Combined Cortical Thickness Congenitally Corrected Transposition; Controlled Cord Traction; Coronary Care Team; Cranial Computerized Tomography

CCTe–Cathodal Closure Tetanus

CCTGA–Congenitally Corrected Transposition of the Great Arteries

CCT in PET–Crude Coal Tar in Petroleum

CCTP–Coronary Care Training Project

CCU–Cardiac Care Unit; Cherry-Crandell Units; Critical Care Unit; Color Changing Unit

CCUP–Colpocystourethropexy

CCV–CCNU, Cyclophosphamide and Vincristine; Conductivity Cell Volume

CCVB–CCNU, Cyclophosphamide, Vincristine and Bleomycin

CCVPP–Cyclophosphamide, CCNU, Vinblastine, Procarbazine and Prednisone

CCVV–Cyclophosphamide, CCNU, VP-16 and Vincristine

CCVVP–Cyclophosphamide, CCNU, VP-16, Vincristine and Cisplatin

CD–Cadaver Donor; Cardiac Disease; Cardiac Dullness; Cardiovascular Disease; Carrel-Dakin; Cesarean Delivery; Combination Drug; Common Duct; Communicable Disease; Consanguineous Donor; Contact Dermatitis; Contagious Disease; Continuous Drainage; Control Diet; Convulsive Disorder; Convulsive Dose; Crohn's Disease; Cutdown; Curative Dose; Cystic Duct

C&D–Curettage and Desiccation; Cystoscopy and Dilatation

Cd–Cadmium (Chemical symbol); Caudal; Coccygeal; Drug Coefficient

CDA–Completely Denatured Alcohol; Congenital Dyserythropoietic Anemia

CDAI–Crohn's Disease Activity Index

CDB–Cough, Deep Breath

CDC–Calculated Date of Confinement; Cancer Detection Center; Centers for Disease Control

CDCA–Chenodeoxycholic Acid

CDD–Certificate of Disability for Discharge; Chronic Disabling Dermatosis

CDDP–Cis-diamminedichloroplatin (Cisplatin)

CDE–Canine Distemper Encephalitis; Common Duct Exploration

CDH–Chronic Daily Headache; Congenital Diaphragmatic Hernia; Congenital Dislocation of Hip

CDLE–Chronic Discoid Lupus Erythematosus

CDP–Collagenase-Digestible Protein; Continuous Distending Pressure; Coronary Drug Project

CDPG–Coronary Drug Project Group

CDS–Chemical Data Systems

CDT–Carbon Dioxide Therapy; Certified Dental Technician

CDYN–Dynamic Compliance of the Lung

CE–California Encephalitis; Cardiac Emergency; Cardiac Enlargement; Cardioesophageal; Central Episiotomy; Cholera Exotoxin; Clinical Emphysema; Conjugated Estrogens; Contrast Echocardiology; Cytopathic Effect

Ce–Cerium (Chemical symbol)

CEA–Carcinoembryonic Antigen; Carotid Endarterectomy

CEBV–Chronic Epstein-Barr Virus

CEC–Ciliated Epithelial Cells

CECT–Contrast Enhancement Computed Tomography

CED–Council on Education for the Deaf

CEI–Continuous Extravascular Infusion

CEJ–Cardioesophageal Junction

cej–Cement-Enamel Junction

CELF–Clinical Evaluation of Language Functions

CELI–Carrow Elicited Language Inventory

CELO–Chicken-Embryo-Lethal-Orphan Virus

CEM–Conventional-Transmission Electron Microscope

C-E Mixture–Chloroform-Ether Mixture

CEN–Certification for Emergency Nursing

CEP–Congenital Erythropoietic Porphyria; Continuing Education Program; Cortical Evoked Potential; Countercurrent Electrophoresis; Cyclophosphamide, Cisplatin and VP-16

CEPH–Cephalic; Cephalosporin

CER–Conditioned Emotional Response

CE&R–Central Episiotomy and Repair

CERA–Cortical Evoked Response Audiometry

CERD–Chronic End-stage Renal Disease

CES–Central Excitatory State; Cognitive Environmental Stimulation

CESD–Cholesterol Ester Storage Disease

CF–Calibration Factor; Cancer-free; Carbon-filtered; Cardiac Failure; Cephalothin; Chiari-Frommel Syndrome; Christmas Factor; Contractile Force; Coronary Flow; Count Fingers; Cystic Fibrosis

C&F–Curettage and Electrodessication

Cf–Californium (Chemical symbol)

CFA–Common Femoral Artery; Complete Freund Adjuvant

CFAC–Complement-Fixing Antibody Consumption

CFD–Concern for the Dying

CFF–Critical Flicker Frequency; Cystic Fibrosis Foundation

CFI–Chemotactic Factor Inactivator

CFM–Close-Fitting Mask

CFP–Cerebral Fluid Protein; Chronic False-Positive; Cyclo-phosphamide, 5-Fluorouracil and Prednisone; Cystic Fibrosis of the Pancreas; Cystic Fibrosis Protein

CFS–Cancer Family Syndrome; Contoured Femoral Stem; Cystic Fibrosis Society

CFT–Complement Fixation Test

CFU–Colony Forming Unit

CFX–Circumflex Artery

CG–Cardio-green; Cholecystogram; Chorionic Gonadotropin; Chronic Glomerulonephritis; Colloidal Gold; Control Group

CGB–Chronic Gastrointestinal Bleeding

CGD–Chronic Granulomatous Disease; Commissural Gastric Driver

CGH–Chorionic Gonadotropic Hormone

CGI–Carbimazole; Clinical Global Impression

CGL–Chronic Granulocytic Leukemia; Correction with Glasses

CGM–Central Gray Matter

CGN–Chronic Glomerulonephritis

CGNB–Composite Ganglioneuroblastoma

CG/OQ–Cerebral Glucose Oxygen Quotient

CGP–Chorionic Growth Hormone Prolactin; Circulating Granulocyte Pool

CGS–Catgut Suture

CGT–Chorionic Gonadotropin

CGTT–Cortisol Glucose Tolerance Test

CH–Cluster Headache; Crown-Heel Length

C&H–Cocaine and Heroin

CHA–Chronic Hemolytic Anemia; Congenital Hypoplastic Anemia

CHAD–Cyclophosphamide, Adriamycin, Cisplatin and Hexamethylmelamine

CHAI–Continuous Hepatic Artery Infusion

CHANCE–Coalition for Handicapped Children's Education

CHAP-S–Cyclophosphamide, Hexamethylmelamine, Adriamycin and Cisplatin

CHB–Complete Heart Block

CHBA–Congenital Heinz Body Hemolytic Anemia

CHD–Chediak-Higashi Disease; Childhood Disease; Common Hepatic Duct; Congenital Heart Disease; Congestive Heart Disease; Coronary Heart Disease; Cyclophosphamide, Hexamethyl-melamine and Cisplatin

CHD-R–Cyclophosphamide, Hexamethylmelamine and Cisplatin and Radiotherapy

CHF–Chronic Heart Failure; Congestive Heart Failure; Crimean Hemorrhagic Fever

CHFV–Combined High Frequency of Ventilation

CHH–Cartilage-Hair Hypoplasia

CHI–Closed Head Injury; Creatinine Height Index

CHL–Chlorambucil; Chloramphenicol

CHN–Carbon, Hydrogen, Nitrogen; Central Hemorrhagic Necrosis; Child Neurology

CHO–Carbohydrate; Cyclophosphamide, Adriamycin and Oncovin

CHOB–Cyclophosphamide, Hydroxydaunorubicin, Oncovin and Bleomycin

CHOP–Cyclophosphamide, Hydroxydaunorubicin, Oncovin and Prednisone

CHOPBLEO–Cyclophosphamide, Hydroxydaunorubicin, Oncovin, Prednisone and Bleomycin

CHOR–Cyclophosphamide, Hydroxydaunorubicin, Vincristine and Radiotherapy

CHP–Child Psychiatry; Comprehensive Health Planning

ChP–Chest Physician

CHRS–Congenital Hereditary Retinoschisis; Cerebrohepatorenal Syndrome

CHS–Chediak-Higashi Syndrome; Compression Hip Screw

CHSD–Children's Health Services Division

CHT–Closed Head Trauma

CHU–Closed Head Unit

CHVP–Cyclophosphamide, Hydroxydaunorubicin, VM-26 and Prednisone

CI–Cardiac Index; Cardiac Insufficiency; Cephalic Index; Cerebral Infarction; Cesium Implant; Chemotherapeutic Index; Clinical Investigation; Clonus Index; Cochlear Implant; Coefficient of Intelligence; Color Index; Complete Iridectomy; Coronary Insufficiency; Crystalline Insulin; Cytotoxic Index

CIA–CCNU, Isophosphamide and Adriamycin; Chronic Idiopathic Anhidrosis; Chymo-trypsin Inhibitor Activity

CIAED–Collagen-induced Autoimmune Ear Disease

CIB–Cytomegalic Inclusion Bodies

CIBD–Chronic Inflammatory Bowel Disease

CIBHA–Congenital Inclusion Body Hemolytic Anemia

CIC–Cardiac Inhibitory Center; Circulating Immune Complexes

CICE–Combined Intracapsular Cataract Extraction

CICS–Adriamycin, VM-26, Cyclophosphamide and Prednisone

CICU–Cardiac Intensive Care Unit; Cardiovascular Inpatient Care Unit

CID–Cytomegalic Inclusion Disease

CIDP–Chronic Inflammatory Demyelinating Polyradiculoneuropathy

CIDS–Cellular Immunity Deficiency Syndrome; Continuous Insulin Delivery System

CIE–Countercurrent Immunoelectrophoresis

CIEP–Counterimmunoelectrophoresis

CIF–Cartilage Induction Factor; Cloning Inhibiting Factor

CIFC–Council for the Investigation of Fertility Control

cigM–Cytoplasmic Immunoglobulin M

CIH–Carbohydrate-Induced Hyperglycemia; Certificate in Industrial Health; Children in Hospitals

CIIS–Cattell Infant Intelligence Scale

CIM–Cortically Induced Movement

CIN–Cervical Intraepithelial Neoplasia; Chronic Interstitial Nephritis

CIOMS–Council for International Organizations of Medical Sciences
CIS–Cancer Information Service; Carcinoma in Situ; Central Inhibitory State
CISCA–Cisplatin, Cytoxan and Adriamycin
cis-DDP–Diamminedichloroplatinum
CIT–Combined Intermittent Therapy
CIU–Chronic Idiopathic Urticaria
CIXU–Constant Infusion Excretory Urogram
CJD–Creutzfeldt-Jakob Disease
CJR–Centric Jaw Relationship
CK–Creatine Kinase; Choline Kinase; Cytokinin
CKC–Cold Knife Conization
CL–Cholesterol-Lecithin; Chronic Leukemia; Corpus Luteum; Lung Compliance
CLA–Cervicolinguoaxial; Cyclic Lysine Anhydride; Community Living Arrangements;
Clinical Laboratory Assistant
CLAS–Congenital Localized Absence of Skin
CLB–Chlorambucil
CLBBB–Complete Left Bundle-Branch Block
CLC–Cork Leather and Celastic
CL/CP–Cleft Lip and Cleft Palate
CLD–Chronic Liver Disease; Chronic Lung Disease
CLE–Centrilobular Emphysema
CLED–Cystine-Lactose Electrolyte Deficient
CLF–Cholesterol-Lecithin Flocculation
CLH–Chronic Lobular Hepatitis
CLIP–Corticotropin-like Intermediate Lobe Peptide
CLL–Cholesterol-Lowering Lipid; Chronic Lymphatic Leukemia; Chronic Lymphocytic Leukemia
CLLE–Columnar-lined Lower Esophagus
CLMN–Complete Lower Motor Neuron

CLO–Cod Liver Oil

CL&P–Cleft Lip and Palate

ClP–Clinical Pathology

CLR–Chloride Test

CLSL–Chronic Lymphosarcoma

CLT–Chronic Lymphocytic Thyroiditis; Clot-lysis Time; Total Lung Compliance

CM–California Mastitis Test; Capreomycin; Cardiac Monitor; Cardiomyopathy; Chick-Martin; Chloroquine-mepacrine; Chondromalacia; Circular Muscle; Cochlear Micro-phonic; Common Migraine; Congenital Malformation; Congestive Myocardiopathy; Continuous Murmur; Contrast Media; Copulatory Mechanism; Costal Margin; Culture Media

Cm–Curium (Chemical Symbol)

CMB–Carbolic Methylene Blue; Central Midwives' Board

CMBBT–Cervical Mucous Basal Body Temperature

CMC–Carpometacarpal; Cell-mediated Cytolysis; Chloramphenicol; Chronic Mucocutaneous Moniliasis; Cyclophosphamide, Methotrexate and CCNU

CMD–Childhood Muscular Dystrophy

CME–Continuing Medical Education; Cystic Macular Edema; Cystoid Macular Edema

CMF–Chondromyxoid Fibroma; Cortical Magnification Factor; Cyclophosphamide, Methotrexate and 5-Fluorouracil

CMF-BLEO–Cyclophosphamide, Methotrexate, 5-Fluorouracil and Bleomycin

CMF-FLU–Cyclophosphamide, Methotrexate, 5-Fluorouracil and Fluoxymesterone

CMFH–Cyclophosphamide, Methotrexate, 5-Fluorouracil and Hydroxyurea

CMFP–Cyclophosphamide, Methotrexate, 5-Fluorouracil and Prednisone

CMFVP–Cyclophosphamide, Methotrexate, 5-Fluorouracil, Vincristine and Prednisone

CMFP-VA–Cyclophosphamide, Methotrexate, 5-Fluorouracil, Prednisone, Vincristine and Adriamycin

CMF-TAM–Cyclophosphamide, Methotrexate, 5-Fluorouracil and Tamoxifen

CMFV–Cyclophosphamide, Methotrexate, 5-Fluorouracil and Vincristine

CMFVP–Cyclophosphamide, Methotrexate, 5-Fluorouracil, Vincristine and Prednisone

CMG–Cystometrogram

CMGN–Chronic Membranous Glomerulonephritis

CMH–Congenital Malformation of the Heart

CMHC–Community Mental Health Center

CMI–Carbohydrate Metabolism Index; Chronic Mesenteric Ischemia

CMID–Cytomegalic Inclusion Disease

CMJ–Carpometacarpal Joint

CMK–Congenital Multicystic Kidney

CML–Cell-Mediated Lympholysis; Chronic Myelocytic Leukemia; Chronic Myelogenous Leukemia

CMM–Cutaneous Malignant Melanoma

CMMT–Columbia Mental Maturity Test

CMN–Cystic Medial Necrosis

CMN-AA–Cystic Medial Necrosis of the Ascending Aorta

CMO–Cardiac Minute Output; Comfort Measures Only; Chief Medical Officer

CMoL–Chronic Monoblastic Leukemia; Chronic Monocytic Leukemia

C-MOPP–Cyclophosphamide, Nitrogen Mustard, Vincristine, Procarbazine and Prednisone

CMOR–Craniomandibular Orthopedic Repositioning Device

CMP–Cardiomyopathy; CCNU, Methotrexate and Procarbazine; Chondromalacia Patellae

CMPF–Cyclophosphamide, Methotrexate, Prednisone and 5-Fluorouracil

CMR–Cerebral Metabolic Rate; Crude Mortality Ratio

CMRG–Cerebral Metabolic Rate of Glucose

CMRNG–Chromosomally Resistant Neisseria Gonorrheae

CMRO–Cerebral Metabolic Rate of Oxygen

CMRR–Common Mode Rejection Ratio

CMS–Cervical Mucous Solution; Chromosome Modification Site; Circulation, Motion and Sensation; Circulatory, Musculatory and Sensory; Click Murmur Syndrome; Clyde Mood Scale; Conflict Management Survey

CMSS–Circulation, Motor Ability, Sensation and Swelling

CMSUA–Clean Midstream Urinalysis

CMT–California Mastitis Test; Certified Medical Transcriptionist; Cervical Motion Tenderness; Current Medical Terminology

CMV–Cool Mist Vaporizer; Continuous Mechanical Ventilation; Cytomegalovirus

CN–Caudate Nucleus; Charge Nurse; Child Nutrition; Cochlear Nursing; Cranial Nerve

CNA–Chart not Available

CNB–Cutting Needle Biopsy

CNC–Clear, no Creamy Layer

CNE–Chronic Nervous Exhaustion

CNF–Cyclophosphamide, Mitoxantrone and Fluorouracil

CNH–Central Neurogenic Hyperpnea; Community Nursing Home

CNHD–Congenital Nonspherocytic Hemolytic Disease

CNM–Certified Nurse-Midwife

CNMT–Certified Nuclear Medicine Technologist

CNP–Continuous Negative Pressure

CNR–Council of National Representatives

CNS–Central Nervous System; Clinical Nurse Specialist

CNSHA–Congenital Nonspherocytic Hemolytic Leukemia

CNT–Could Not test

CNV–Colistimethate, Nystatin and Vancomycin; Conative Negative Variation; Contigent Negative Variation

CO–Carbon Monoxide; Cardiac Output; Castor Oil; Centric Occlusion; Cervicoaxial; Choline Oxidase; Corneal Opacity; Corpus; Crossover

Co–Cobalt (chemical symbol)

CoA–Coarctation of the Aorta; Coenzyme A

COAD–Chronic Obstructive Airway Disease; Chronic Obstructive Arterial Disease

COAG–Chronic Open-Angle Glaucoma

COAP–Cyclophosphamide, Vincristine, Cytarabine and Prednisone

COAP-BLEO–Cyclophosphamide, Vincristine, Cytarabine, Prednisone and Bleomycin

COB–Cisplatin, Oncovin and Bleomycin

COBS–Cesarean-Obtained Barrier-sustained

COBT–Chronic Obstruction of the Biliary Tract

COC–Cathodal Opening Clonus; Cathodal Opening Contraction; Coccygeal; Combination-type Oral Contraceptive

COCL–Cathodal Opening Clonus

COD–Cause of Death; Codeine; Condition on Discharge

COEAMRA–Council on Education of the American Medical Record Association

COEPS–Cortically Originating Extrapyramidal Symptoms

COG–Central Oncology Group; Cognitive

COGTT–Cortisone-Primed Oral Glucose Tolerance Test

COHB–Craboxyhemoglobin

COLD–Chronic Obstructive Lung Disease

COLD A–Cold Agglutinin Titer

COM–College of Osteopathic Medicine; Cyclophosphamide, Oncovin and MeCCNU

COMA-A–Cyclophosphamide, Oncovin, Methotrexate, Adriamycin, Citrovorum Factor and Cytosine Arabinoside

COMB–Cyclophosphamide, Oncovin, MeCCNU and Bleomycin

COMBAP–Cytoxan, Oncovin, Methotrexate, Bleomycin, Adriamycin and Prednisone

COMe–Cytoxan, Oncovin and Methotrexate

COMF–Cyclophosphamide, Oncovin, Methotrexate and 5-Fluorouracil

COMLA–Cyclophosphamide, Oncovin, Methotrexate and Ara-C

COMP–Cyclophosphamide, Oncovin, Methotrexate and Procarbazine

COMT–Catechol-O-Methyl Transferase; Certified Ophthalmic Medical Assistant

CONPADRI I–Cyclophosphamide, Vincristine, Doxorubicin and Melphalan

CONPADRI II–Cyclophosphamide, Vincristine, Doxorubicin, Melphalan and High Dose Methotrexate

CONPADRI III–Cyclophosphamide, Vincristine, Doxorubicin, Melphalan and Intensified Doxorubicin

CONPADRI V–Cyclophosphamide, Vincristine, Melphalan, Adriamycin and Methotrexate

COOD–Chronic Obstructive Outflow Disease

COP–Change of Plaster; Cicatricial Ocular Pemphigoid; Colloid Osmotic Pressure; Cyclophosphamide, Oncovin and Prednisone

COPA–Cyclophosphamide, Oncovin, Adriamycin and Prednisone

COPAC–CCNU, Oncovin, Prednisone, Adriamycin and Cyclophosphamide

COPB–Cyclophosphamide, Oncovin, Prednisone and Bleomycin

COP-BLAM–Cyclophosphamide, Oncovin, Prednisone, Procarbazine, Bleomycin and Adriamycin

COPD–Chronic Obstructive Pulmonary Disease

COPE–Chronic Obstructive Pulmonary Emphysema

COPI–California Occupational Preference Inventory

COPP–Cyclophosphamide, Oncovin, Procarbazine and Prednisone

COR–Cardiac Output Recorder; Conditioned Orienting Response

CORA–Conditioned Orientation Reflex Audiometry

CORD–Chronic Obstructive Respiratory Disease

CORT–Certified Operating Room Technician

COS–Chief of Staff; Clinical Orthopedic Society

COT–Cathodal Opening Tetanus; Content of Thought; Contralateral Optic Tectum

COTA–Certified Occupational Therapy Assistant

COU–Cardiac Observation Unit

COWAT–Controlled Oral Word Association Test

COWS–Cold to Opposite, Warm to Same

COX–Cast-Off X-Ray

CP–Capillary Pressure; Cerebellopontine; Cerebral Palsy; Cerebropontine; Certified Prothetist; Chest Pains; Child Psychiatry; Chloroquine and Primaquine; Chondromalacia Patella; Chronic Pain; Chronic Pyelonephritis; Cisplatin; Cleft Palate; Clinical Pathology; Closing Pressure; Cochlear Potential; Color Perception; Compressed Tablet; Constant Pressure; Coracoid Process; Cor Pulmonale; Creatine Phosphate; Creatine Phosphokinase; Cyclophosphamide

C&P–Cystoscopy and Pyelography

Cp–Chickenpox

CPA–Cardiopulmonary Arrest; Carotid Phonoangiography; Cerebellar Pontine Angle; Circulating Platelet Aggregate; Costophrenic Angle; Cyclophosphamide

CPAF–Chlorpropamide-Alcohol Flush

CPAP–Constant Positive Air Pressure; Continuous Positive Air Pressure

CPB–Cardiopulmonary Bypass

CPC–Cerebral Palsy Clinic; Chronic Passive Congestion; Circumferential Pneumatic Compression; Clinical Pathological Conference

CPCL–Congenital Pulmonary Cystic Lymphangiectasis

CPCP–Chronic Progressive Coccidioidal Pneumonitis

CPCR–Cardiopulmonary-Cerebral Resuscitation

CPD–Cephalopelvic Disproportion; Chorioretinopathy and Pituitary Dysfunction; Citrate-Phosphate-Dextrose; Contagious Pustular Dermatitis

CPDA-1–Citrate-Phosphate-Dextrose-Adenine

CPDD–Calcium Pyrophosphate Deposition Disease

CPE–Cardiogenic Pulmonary Edema; Chronic Pulmonary Emphysema; Cytopathic effect

CPF–Clot-Promoting Factor

CPG–Capillary Blood Gases

CPGN–Chronic Progressive Glomerulonephritis

CPH–Chronic Persistant Hepatitis

CPH 5W–Cutter Protein Hydrolysate Five Percent in Water

CPHA–Committee on Professional and Hospital Activities

CPI–California Psychological Inventory; Cancer Potential Index; Constitutional Psychopathic Inferiority; Coronary Prognostic Index

CPID–Chronic Pelvic Inflammatory Disease

CPIP–Common Peak Developed Isovolumic Pressure

CPK–Creatine Phosphokinase

CPKD–Childhood Polycystic Kidney Disease

CPM–Central Pontine Myelinolysis; Continuous Passive Motion; Counts per Minute; Cycles per Minute; Cyclophosphamide

CPN–Chronic Pyelonephritis

CPOB–Cyclophosphamide, Prednisone, Oncovin and Bleomycin

CPP–Cerebral Perfusion Pressure

CPPB–Constant Positive-Pressure Breathing; Continuous Positive-Pressure Breathing

CPPD–Calcium Pyrophosphate Deposition Disease

CPPV–Continuous Positive-Pressure Ventilation

CPR–Cardiac Pulmonary Reserve; Cardiopulmonary Resuscitation; Centripetal Rub; Cerebral Cortex Perfusion Rate

CPRD–Committee on Prosthetics Research and Development

CPS–Chloroquine, Pyrimethamine and Sulfisoxazole; Clinical Performance Score; Complex Partial Seizure; Constitutional Psychopathic State; Cardiopulmonary Support System

CPT–Carotid Pulse Tracing; Chest Physiotherapy; Ciliary Particle Transport; Clinical Pharmacokinetics Team; Cold Pressure Test; Concentration Performance Test; Conti-nuous Performance Test; Current Procedural Terminology

CPTH–Chronic Post-Traumatic Headache; C-Terminal Parathyroid Hormone

CPUE–Chest Pain of Unknown Etiology

CPZ–Chlorpromazine

CR–Calculus Removal; Cardiac Rehabilitation; Cardiorespiratory; Cartilage Residue; Centric Relation; Chest Roentgenogram; Clinical Record; Clinical Research; Closed Reduction; Clot Retraction; Colon Resection; Complete Remission; Conditioned Reflex; Conditioned Response; Controlled Release; Conversion Ratio; Crown-Rump

Cr–Chromium (Chemical Symbol)

CRA–Central Retinal Artery; Chinese Restaurant Asthma

CRAO–Central Retinal Artery Occlusion

CRBBB–Complete Right Bundle-branch Block

CRC–Calomel, Rhubarb, Colocynth; Cardiac Reconditioning Center; Cardiovascular Reflex Conditioning; Colorectal Cancer; Crisis Resolution Center

CrCl–Creatinine Clearance

CRCS–Cardiovascular Reflex Conditioning System

CRD–Chronic Renal Disease; Chronic Respiratory Disease; Crown-Rump Distance

CRE–Cumulative Radiation Effect

CREST–Calcinosis, Raynaud's Phenomenon, Esophageal Dysmotility, Sclerodactyly and Telangiectasia

CRF–Chronic Renal Failure; Chronic Respiratory Failure; Corticotropin-releasing Factor

CRG–Cardiorespirogram

CRH–Corticotropin-Releasing Hormone

CRI–Chronic Renal Insufficiency; Cold Running Intelligibility; Cross-Reactive Idiotype

CRL–Crown-Rump Length

CRNA–Certified Registered Nurse Anesthetist

CRNP–Certified Registered Nurse Practitioner

CRO–Cathode Ray Oscillograph; Cathode Ray Oscilloscope; Centric Relation Occlusion

CROP–Cyclophosphamide, Rubidazone, Oncovin and Prednisone

CROPAM–Cyclophosphamide, Rubidazone, Oncovin, Prednisone, L-asparaginase and Methotrexate

CROS–Contralateral Routing of Signal

CRRT–Certified Respiratory Therapy Technician

CRS–Central Supply Room; Colon-Rectal Surgery; Congenital Rubella Syndrome

CRST–Calcification, Raynaud's Phenomenon, Scleroderma and Telangiectasia

CRT–Cardiac Resuscitation Team; Cathode Ray Tube; Central Reaction Time; Complex Reaction Timer

CRTX–Cast Removed, Take to X-ray

CRU–Crisis Resolution Center; Clinical Research Unit

CRV–Central Retinal Vein

CRVO–Central Retinal Vein Occlusion

CRYST–Crystal Examination Screen

CS–Carcinoid Syndrome; Cardiogenic Shock; Carotid Sheath; Carotid Sinus; Cat Scratch; Celiac Sprue; Central Supply; Cerebrospinal;

Cervical Spine; Cesarean Section; Chemical Sympathectomy; Chronic Schizophrenia; Cigarette Smoke; Cockayne's Syndrome; Collet-Sicard Syndrome; Completed Stroke; Completed Suicide; Concentrated Strength; Conditioned Stimulus; Congenital Syphilis; Conjunctiva-Sclera; Consciousness; Contact Sensitivity; Continuous Stripping; Coronary Sclerosis; Coronary Sinus; Corpus Striatum; Cortical Spoking; Corticosteroid; Current Strength; Curschmann-Steinert; Cushing's Syndrome

Cs–Cesium (Chemical Symbol)

CSA–Colon-Specific Antigens

CSAP–Colon-Specific Antigen Protein

CSBF–Coronary Sinus Blood Flow

CSC–Central Serous Choroidopathy; Collagen Sponge Contraceptive; Cryogenic Storage Container

CSCD–Center for Sickle Cell Disease

CSD–Cat Scratch Disease; Conditionally Streptomycin Dependent; Cortically Spreading Depression

CSE–Cross-section Echocardiography

CSF–Cerebrospinal Fluid

CSH–Carotid Sinus Hypersensitivity; Chronic Subdural Hematoma; Cortical Stromal Hyper-plasia

CSICU–Cardiac Surgical Intensive Care Unit

CSII–Continuous Subcutaneous Insulin Infusion

CSLU–Chronic Stasis Leg Ulcer

CSM–Cerebrospinal Meningitis; Circulation, Sensation, Movement; Corn-Soy Milk

CSMB–Center for the Study of Multiple Births

CSMMG–Chartered Society of Message and Medical Gymnastics

CSN–Carotid Sinus Nerve

CSOM–Chronic Serous Otitis Media; Chronic Suppurative Otitis Media

CSP–Cavum Septum Pellucidum; Chartered Society of Physiotherapy; Cooperative Statistical Program; Criminal Sexual Psychopath

CSR–Central Supply Room; Cheynes-Stokes Respiration; Corrective Septorhinoplasty; Cortical Secretion Rate

CSS–Carotid Sinus Stimulation; Central Sterile Supply; Chewing, Sucking, Swallowing; Chronic Subclinical Scurvy

CST–Cardiac Stress Test; Cavernous Sinus Thrombosis; Certified Surgical Technologist; Contraction Stress Test; Convulsive Shock Therapy; Cosyntropin Stimulation Test

CSU–Cardiac Surveillance Unit; Cardiovascular Surgery Unit; Central Statistical Unit

CT–Cardiothoracic; Cardiovascular Technologist; Carotid Tracing; Carpal Tunnel; Cerebral Thrombosis; Cervical Traction; Chest Tube; Circulating Time; Classic Technique; Clotting Time; Coagulation Time; Coated Tablet; Collecting Tubule; Computed Tomography; Connective Tissue; Continue Treatment; Continuous-flow Tub; Contraceptive Technique; Contraction Time; Controlled Temperature; Coombs' Test; Corneal Thickness; Corneal Transplant; Coronary Thrombosis; Corrected Transposition; Corrective Therapist; Cytotechnologist

CTA–Clear to Auscultation; Computerized Tomoangiography; Cyanotrimethyl-Androsterone

Cta–Catamenia

CTAC–Carrow Test for Auditory Comprehension; Cancer Treatment Advisory Committee

CTAP–Connective Tissues Activating Peptides

CTAT–Computerized Transaxial Tomography

CTB–Ceased to Breath

CTC–Chlortetracycline

CTCL–Cutaneous T-Cell Lymphoma

ctCO2–Concentration of Total Carbon Dioxide

CTD–Carpal Tunnel Decompression; Chest Tube Drainage; Congenital Thymic Dysplasia; Convalescent Training Depot
CT&DB–Cough, Turn and Deep Breath
CTEM–Conventional Transmission Electron Microscope
CTF–Cancer Therapy Facility; Colorado Tick Fever; Cytotoxic Factor
CTG–Cardiotocography
CTIU–Cardiac/Thoracic Intensive Care Unit
CTL–Cytologic Thymus-Dependent Lymphocyte
ctl–Contact Lens
CTM–Chlor-Trimeton
CTMM–Computed Tomographic Metrizamide Myelography
CT/MPR–Computed Tomography with Multiplanar Reconstructions
cTNM–Clinical-Diagnostic Staging of Cancer
CTP–Comprehensive Treatment Plan
CTS–Carpal Tunnel Syndrome; Computerized Tomographic Scanner
CTSP–Called to See Patient
CTT–Compressed Tablet Titurate; Computed Tansaxial Tomography
CTU–Cardiac/Thoracic Unit; Centigrade Thermal Unit
CTW–Central Terminal of Wilson
CTX–Cefotaxime; Cerebrotendinous; Cytoxan; Xanthomatosis
CTXN–Contraction
CTZ–Chemoreceptor Trigger Zone; Chlorthiazide
CU–Cause Unknown; Chymotrypsin Unit; Clinical Unit; Color Unit; Convalescent Unit
Cu–Copper (Chemical Symbol)
CUC–Chronic Ulcerative Colitis
CUD–Cause Undetermined
CUG–Cystidine-Uridine-Guanidine; Cystourethrogram
CUP–Care Unit Program
CURN–Conduct and Utilization of Research in Nursing
CUS–Chronic Undifferentiated Schizophrenia
CUSA–Cavitron Ultrasonic Surgical Aspirator

CV–Cardiovascular; Central Venous; Cerebrovascular; Cervical Vertebra; Closed Vitrectomy; Closing Volume; Color Vision; Concentrated Volume; Conjugata Vera; Conversational Voice; Corpuscular Volume; Costovertebral; Cyclophosphamide and VP-16

CVA–Cardiovascular Accident; Cerebrovascular Accident; Costovertebral Angle; Cyclophos-phamide, Vincristine and Adriamycin

CVAT–Costovertebral Angle Tenderness

CVB–CCNU, Vinblastine and Bleomycin

CVC–Central Venous Catheter

CVCT–Cardiovascular Computerized Tomography

CVD–Cardiovascular Disease; Cerebrovascular Disease; Collagen Vascular Disease; Color-Vision Deviant

CVF–Central Visual Field

CVH–Combined Ventricular Hypertrophy; Common Variable Hypogammaglobulinemia

CVI–Cerebrovascular Insufficiency; Common Variable Immunodeficiency; Continuous Venous Infusion

CVID–Common Variable Immune Deficiency

CVM–Cardiovascular Monitor; Cyclophosphamide, Vincristine and Methotrexate

CVO–Central Vein Occlusion; Conjugata Vera Obstetrica

CVOD–Cerebrovascular Obstructive Disease

CVP–Central Venous Pressure; Cerebrovascular Profile; Cyclophos-phamide, Vincristine andPrednisolone; Cyclophosphamide, Vincristine and Prednisone

CVPP–CCNU, Vinblastine, Procarbazine and Prednisone

CVR–Cardiovascular-Renal Disease; Cardiovascular-Respiratory; Cephalic Vasomotor Response; Cerebrovascular Resistance

CVRD–Cardiovascular Renal Disease

CVRI–Coronary Vascular Resistance Index

CVS–Cardiovascular Surgery; Cardiovascular System; Chorionic Villus Sampling

CVUG–Cystoscopy and Voiding Urethrogram

CW–Cardiac Work; Chest Wall; Children's Ward; Clockwise; Continuous Wave; Crutch Walking

CWBTS–Capillary Whole Blood True Sugar

CWD–Continuous-Wave Doppler

CWE–Cotton-Wool Exudates

CWI–Cardiac Work Index

CWMS–Color, Warmth, Movement, Sensation

CWOP–Childbirth Without Pain

CWP–Centimeters of Water Pressure; Childbirth Without Pain; Coal Workers' Pneumoconiosis

CWPEA–Childbirth Without Pain Education Association

CWS–Child Welfare Service; Cold-Water Soluble; Cotton-Wool Spots

CWT–Cold Water Treatment

CX–Cervix; Chest X-ray; Cyclophosphamide

cx–Cylinder Axis

CxMT–Cervical Motion Tenderness

CXR–Chest Roentgenogram

CYA–Cyclosporine

CYC–Cyclophosphamide

CY-VA-DACT–Cyclophosphamide, Vincristine, Adriamycin and Actinomycin D

CYVADIC–Cyclophosphamide, Vincristine, Adriamycin and Dacarbazine

CY-VA-DIC–Cyclophosphamide, Vincristine, Adriamycin and DTIC (Dacarbazine)

CZ–Carzinophilin; Cefazolin

CZI–Crystalline Zinc Insulin

D

D–Cholecalciferol; Dead; Dental; Deuterium; Diameter; Diarrhea; Diathermy; Diffusion Constant; Diopter; Disease; Distal; Dopamine; Dorsal; Dose; Duodenum; Drive State; Dwarf; Drug; Difference

d–Day; Density; Deoxyribose; Diastolic; Duration; Dyne; Dorsal

DA–Daunomycin and Cytosine Arabinoside; Decubitus Angina; Degenerative Arthritis; Delayed Action; Dental Assistant; Developmental Age; Diploma in Anesthetics; Direct Admission; District Administrator; Dopamine; Drug Addict; Ductus Arteriosus

DAB–Dysrhythmic Aggressive Behavior

DACA–Drug Abuse Control Amendments

DAD–Dispense as Directed; Drug Administration Device

DADDS–Diacetyl Diaminodiphenylsulfone

DADPS–Diphenylsulfone

DAE–Driving Air Embolism

DAF–Delayed Auditory Feedback; Draw-A-Family Test

DAG–Dianhydrogalacitol

DAH–Disordered Action of the Heart

DAI–Diffuse Axonal Injury

DANA–Drug-Induced Antinuclear Antibodies

DAP–Diaminopimelic Acid; Direct Agglutination Pregnancy Test; Draw-A-Person Test

DAP I–Diahydrogalactitol, Adriamycin and Cisplatin

DAP II–Diahydrogalactitol, Adriamycin and High Dose Cisplatin

DAPRU–Drug Abuse Prevention Resource Unit

DAPST–Denver Auditory Phoneme Sequencing Test

DAPT–Direct Agglutination Pregnancy Test

DARTS–Drug and Alcohol Rehabilitation Testing System

DAS–Data Acquisition System

DASA–Distal Articular Set Angle

DASI–Developmental Activities Screening Inventory

DAT–Daunorubicin, Cytarabine and Thioguanine; Delayed Action Tablet; Dementia of the Alzheimer's Type; Dental Admission Test; Diet as Tolerated; Differential Agglutination Titer; Differential Aptitude Test; Diptheria Antitoxin; Direct Agglutination Test; Disaster Action Team

DAW–Dispense as Written

DB–Baudelocque's Diameter (External Conjugate Diameter of Pelvis); Date of Birth; Deep Breath; Distobuccal

Db–Diabetic

dB–Decibel

DB&C–Deep Breathing and Coughing

DBCL–Dilute Blood Clot Lysis Method

DBE–Deep Breathing Exercise

DBED–Penicillin G Benzathine

DBH–Dacarbazine, Carmustine and Hydroxyurea

DBI–Development at Birth Index; Phenethylbiguanide

DBIL–Direct Bilirubin

DBIP–Discrimination by Identification of Pictures

DBK–Diabetic Management; Dibromomannitol

DBM–Diabetic Management; Dibromannitol

DBO–Distobucco-occlusal

DBP–Diastolic Blood Pressure; Distobuccopulpal

DBQ–Debrisoquin

DBR–Direct Bilirubin

DBS–Deep Brain Stimulation; Denis Browne Splint; Diminished Breath Sounds; Despeciated Bovine Serum

DBV–Dacarbazine, Carmustine and Vincristine

DBW–Desireable Body Weight

DC–Daily Census; Diagnostic Center; Diagonal Conjugate; Digit Copying; Direct and Consensual; Distocervical; Donor's Cells

D&C–Dilatation and Curettage; Dilation and Curettage; Drugs and Cosmetics

DCA–Dichloroacetic Acid

DC&B–Dilation, Curettage and Biopsy

DCC–Day Care Center

DCCMP–Daunomycin, Cyclocytidine, 6-Mercaptopurine and Prednisolone

DCF–Direct Centrifugal Flotation

DCFM–Doppler Color Flow Mapping

DCH–Delayed Cutaneous Hypersensitivity

DCI–Dichloroisoproterenol

DCM–Dichloromethotrexate

DCMP–Daunomycin, Cytosine Arabinoside, 6-Mercaptopurine and Prednisolone

DCMXT–Dichloromethtrexate

DCN–Delayed Conditional Necrosis; Dorsal Cutaneous Nerve

DCO–Diffusing Capacity of Carbon Monoxide

DCP–Decentralized Pharmacy; Dynamic Compression Plate

DCR–Dacryocystorhinostomy; Delayed Cutaneous Reaction; Direct Cortical Response

DCS–Dense Canalicular System; Dorsal Column Stimulator

DCSA–Double Contrast Shoulder Arthrography

DCT–Deep Chest Therapy; Diastolic Control Team; Direct Coomb's Test; Distal Convoluted Tubule

DCTM–Delay Computer Tomographic Myelography

DCV–Dacarbazine, Lomustine and Vincristine

DD–Dangerous Drug; Degenerative Disease; Dependent Drainage; Developmental Disability; Died of Disease; Differential Diagnosis; Disk Diameter; Down Drain; Dry Dressing; Duchenne's Dystrophy; Discharged Dead; Developmental Disability

D&D–Diarrhea and Dehydration

DDA–Dangerous Drugs Act

DDAVP–1-Deamino-(8-D-arginine)-vasopressin

DDC–Dangerous Drug Cabinet

DDD–Degenerative Disk Disease; Dense Deposit Disease

DDI–Dressing Dry and Intact

DDIB–Disease Detection Information Bureau

DDO–Diploma in Dental Orthopedics

DDP–Cisplatin

DDR–Diploma in Diagnostic Radiology

DDS–Demos Dropout Scale; Dialysis Disequilibrium Syndrome; Dystrophy-Dystocia Syndrome; Doctor of Dental Science; Doctor of Dental Surgery

DDSO–Dapsone

DDST–Denver Developmental Screening Test

DDT–Dichlorodiphenyltrichloroethane; Ductus Deferens Tumor

Ddx–Differential Diagnosis

DE–Dentistry; Deprived Eye; Drug Equivalent; Dream Elements; Drug Evaluation; Duration of Ejection

D&E–Diet and Elimination; Dilatation and Evacuation

DEA–Dehydroepiandrosterone; Drug Enforcement Administration

DEBRA–Dystrophic Epidermolysis Bullosa Reasearch Association

DECO–Decreasing Consumption of Oxygen

DED–Date of Expected Delivery; Delayed Erythema Dose

DEEG–Depth Electroencephalogram; Depth Electrography

DEET–Diethyltoluamide

DEF–Decayed, Extracted or Filled

DEHS–Division of Emergency Health Service

DEM–Department of Emergency Medicine

DES–Diethylstilbestrol; Diffuse Esophageal Spasm; Disequilibrium Syndrome; Doctors' Emergency Service

DET–Dimethyltryptamine

DEV–Development; Deviation; Duck Egg Vaccine; Duck Embryo Vaccine

DEVR–Dominant Exudative Vitreoretinopathy

DF–Decapitation Factor; Decayed and Filled; Deferoxamine Mesylate; Deficiency Factor; Degree of Freedom; Dermatology Foundation; Desferrioxamine; Diabetic Father; Dietary Fiber; Disseminated Foci; Distribution Factor; Dorsiflexion

DFA–Diet for Age; Direct Fluorescent Antibody

DFB–Dinitrofluorobenzene; Dysfunctional Uterine Bleeding

DFC–Dry-Filled Capsules

DFD–Defined Formula Diets

DFE–Distal Femoral Epiphysis

DFI–Disease Free Intervals

DFMC–Daily Fetal Movements Record

DFO–Deferoxamine

DFP–Diastolic Filling Period

DFR–Diabetic Floor Routine

DFSP–Dermatofibrosarcoma Protuberans

DFU–Dead Fetus in Utero

DG–Diagnosis; Diastolic Gallop; Distogingival

DGE–Density Gradient Electrophoresis

DGI–Disseminated Gonococcal Infection

DGM–Ductal Glandular Mastectomy

DGO–Diploma in Gynecology and Obstetrics

DGS–Diabetic Glomerulosclerosis

DH–Day Hospital; Delayed Hypersensitivity; Dermatitis Herpetiformis; Developmental History; Diaphragmatic Hernia; Diffuse Histiocytic Lymphoma; Disseminated Histoplasmosis; Dominant Hand; Drug Hypersensitivity

DHA–Dehydroepiandrosterone; Dihydroxyacetone

DHAD–Anthraquinone Dihydrochloride

DHAP–Dihydroxyacetone Phosphate

DHBV–Duck Hepatitis B Virus

DHC–Dehydrocholic Acid

DHE–Dihydroergotamine

DHF–Dengue Hemorrhagic Fever

DHI–Dihydroxyindol

DHIC–Dihydroisocodeine

DHK–Dihydroergocryptine

DHL–Diffuse Histiocytic Lymphoma

DHM–Dihydromorphine

DHO–Dihydroergocornine

DHPG–Gancyclovir

DHR–Delayed Hypersensitivity Reaction

DHS–Department of Human Services; Duration of Hospital Stay; Dynamic Hip Screw

D-5-HS–Dextrose Five Percent in Hartman's Solution

DHSM–Dihydrostreptomycin

DHSS–Dihydrostreptomycin Sulfate

DHT–Theophylline

DHTB–Dihydroteleocidin B

DHTP–Dihydrotestosterone Proprionate

DHZ–Dihydralazine

DI–Deterioration Index; Detrusor Instability; Diabetes Insipidus; Diagnostic Imaging; Distoincisal; Drug Information; Drug Interactions; Dyskaryosis Index; Dyspnea Index

Di–Insulin Dialysance

DIC–Dacarbazine; Different Interference Contrast; Diffuse Intravascular Coagulation; Diffuse Intravascular Coagulopathy; Dimethyl Imidazole Carboxamide; Drug Information Center

DID–Dead of Intercurrent Disease

DIE–Died in Emergency Room; Direct Injection Enthalpimetry

DIG–Digoxin

DIJOA–Diminantly Inherited Juvenile Optic Atrophy

DILD–Diffuse Infiltrative Lung Disease

DILE–Drug-Induced Lupus Erythematosus

DIMOAD–Diabetes Insipidus, Diabetes Mellitus; Optic Atrophy and Deafness Syndrome

DIP–Desquamative Interstitial Pneumonia; Distal Interphalangeal Joint; Drip Infusion Pyelogram; Dual In-Line Package

DIPJ–Distal Interplalangeal Joint

DIS–Diagnostic Interview Scheduled

DISH–Diffuse Idiopathic Skeletal Hyperostosis

DISI–Dorsal Intercalary Segment Instability

DIT–Diiodotyrosine

DIV–Double-inlet Ventricle

DIVA–Digital Intravenous Angiography

DJD–Degenerative Joint Disease

DK–Diseased Kidney

Dk–Diffusion Coefficient

DKA–Diabetic Ketoacidosis

DKB–Deep Knee Bends

DL–Diagnostic Laparoscopy; Diffuse Limen Threshold; Diffuse Lymphoma; Diffusing Capacity of the Lung; Direct Laryngoscopy; Disabled List; Distolingual

DLA–Distolabial

Dlai–Distolabioincisal

DLAP–Distolabiopulpal

DL&B–Direct Laryngoscopy and Bronchoscopy

DLC–Differential Leukocyte Count

DLCO–Diffusing Capacity of the Lungs for Carbon Monoxide

DLE–Discoid Lupus Erythematosus; Disseminated Lupus Erythematosus

DLF–Disabled Living Foundation; Dorsolateral Funiculus

DLI–Distolinguoincisal

DLL–Dihomo-gammalinoleic Acid

DLMP–Date of Last Menstrual Period

DLO–Diploma in Laryngology and Otology; Distolinguo-Occlusal

DLP–Distolinguopulpal

D5LR–Dextrose Five Percent in Lactated Ringer's

DLT–Dihydroepiandrosterone Loading Test

DLVO–Derjaguin-Landau-Verway-Overbeek Theory

DM–Dermatomyositis;   Dextromethorphan;   Diabetes   Mellitus;
    Diabetic Mother; Diastolic Murmur; Diffuse Mixed Lymphoma;
    Diploma in Dermatological Medicine; Doctor of Dental Medicine;
    Dopamine; Diabetes Mellitus

Dm–Diffusing Capacity of the Alveolar Capillary Membrane

DMARD's–Disease Modifying Antirheumatic Drugs

DMC–Demeclocycline

DMCT–Dimethylchlortetracycline

DMCTC–Dimethylchlortetracycline

DMD–Duchenne's Muscular Dystrophy; Doctor of Dental Medicine

DME–Dextromethorphan; Durable Medical Equipment

DMF–Decayed, Missing or Filled

DMFT–Decayed, Missing and Filled Permanent Teeth

DMH–Department of Mental Health

DMHS–Director of Medical and Health Services

DMI–Desipramine; Diagnostic Medical Instruments; Diaphragmatic
    Myocardial Infarct

DMJ–Diploma in Medical Jurisprudence

DMKA–Diabetes Mellitus Ketoacidosis

DML–Diffuse Mixed Lymphoma

DMN–Dorsal Motor Nucleus

DMOOC–Diabetes Mellitus Out of Control

DMRE–Diploma in Medical Radiology and Electrology

DMS–Department of Medicine and Surgery; Dermatomyositis;
    Diagnostic Medical Sonographer; Doctor of Medical Science

DMSA–2,3-Dimercaptosuccinic Acid

DMSLT–Daytime Multiple Sleep Latency Test

DMSO–Dimethyl Sulfoxide

DMU–Dimethanolurea; Dimethyluracil

DMX–Diathermy, Massage and Exercise

DN–Dicrotic Notch; Diploma in Nursing; Diploma in Nutrition

DNA–Deoxyribonucleic Acid; Does Not Apply

DNC–Did Not Come

DND–Died a Natural Death

DNE–Director of Nursing Education; Group D Nonenterococcal Streptococcus

DNI–Do Not Intubate

DNKA–Did Not Keep Appointment

DNR–Daunorubicin; Do Not Report; Do Not Resuscitate

DNS–Deviated Nasal Septum; Diaphragm Nerve Stimulation; Did Not Show; Dysplastic Nevus Syndrome

D5/NS–Dextrose Five Percent in Normal Saline

DNT–Did Not Test

DO–Dissolved Oxygen; Doctor of Ophthalmology; Doctor of Optometry; Doctor of Osteopathy; Doctor's Orders

DOA–Date of Admission; Dead on Arrival

DOAC–Dubois Oleic Albumin Complex

DOA-DRA–Dead on Arrival Despite Resuscitative Attempts

DOAP–Daunorubicin, Oncovin, Adriamycin and Prednisone

DOB–Date of Birth; Dobutamine; Doctor's Order Book

DOC–11-deoxycorticosterone; Diabetes Out of Control; Died of Other Causes

DOCA–Deoxycorticosterone Acetate

DOCG–Deoxycorticosterone Glucoside

DOCs–Deoxycorticoids

DOC-SR–Desoxycorticosterone Secretion Rate

DOD–Date of Death; Dead of Disease; Dissolved Oxygen Deficit

DOE–Date of Examination; Desoxyephedrine Hydrochloride; Dyspnea on Exertion

DOI–Date of Injury; Died of Injuries

DOLV–Double Outlet Left Ventricle

DOM–Dominant

DOMS–Diploma in Ophthalmic Medicine and Surgery; Doctor of Orthopedic Medicine and Surgery

DON–Director of Nursing; Diazo-oxonorleucine

DOOR–Deafness, Onychodystrophy, Osteodystrophy, Retardation

DOPA–Methyldopa; Dopamine

DOPS–Diffuse Obstructive Pulmonary Syndrome

DOVR–Double Outlet Right Ventricle

DOS–Date of Surgery; Doctor of Ocular Science; Doctor of Optical Science

DOSC–Dubois Oleic Serum Complex

DOSS–Dioctyl Sodium Sulfosuccinate; Distal Over-shoulder Strap

DOT–Died on Table; Doppler Ophthalmic Test

DOU–Definitive Observation Unit; Direct Observation Unit

DOV–Discharged on Visit

DP–Deep Pulse; Deltopectoral; Dementia Praecox; Dental Prosthetics; Diastolic Pressure; Diffusion Pressure; Digestible Protein; Dipropionate; Direct Puncture; Directional Preponderance; Displaced Person; Distal Phalanx; Distopulpal; Doctor of Pharmacy; Donor's Plasma; Dorsalis Pedis

DPA–Dextroposition of Aorta

DPC–Delayed Primary Closure; Direct Patient Care; Desaturated Phosphatidylcholine; Discharge Planning Coordinator; Distal Palmar Crease

DPD–Desoxypyridoxine Hydrochloride; Diffuse Pulmonary Disease

DPDL–Diffuse, Poorly Differentiated Lymphoma

DPDLL–Diffuse, Poorly Differentiated, Lymphocytic Lymphoma

DPF–Dental Practitioners' Formulary

DPG–Displacement Placentogram

DPHN–Doctor of Public Health Nursing

DPIF–Drug Product Information File

DPL–Distopulpolingual

DPM–Diploma in Psychological Medicine; Discontinue Previous Medication; Disintegration per Minute; Doctor of Podiatric Medicine; Doctor of Psychiatric Medicine

DPP–Dimethoxyphenyl Penicillin

DPT–Demerol, Phenergen and Thorazine; Dimethyltryptamine; Diphtheria, Pertussis and Tetanus

DPTI–Diastolic Pressure Time Index

DPU–Delayed Pressure Urticaria; Diphenylhydantoin

DQ–Developmental Quotient

DR–Daunorubicin; Delivery Room; Diabetic Retinopathy; Diagnostic Radiology; Dorsal Root

DREZ–Dorsal Root Entry Zone

DRF–Daily Replacement Factor; Deafness Research Foundation; Dose-reduction Factor

DRG–Diagnosis-Related Groups; Dorsal Respiratory Group; Dorsal Root Ganglion

DRI–Direct Rooming In; Discharge Readiness Inventory

DRIC–Dental Research Information Center

DRLS–Del Rio Language Screening

DRME–Division of Research in Medical Education

DRnt–Diagnostic Roentgenology

DRQ–Discomfort Relief Quotient

DS–Dead-air Space; Dehydroepiandrosterone Sulfate; Density Standard; Dental Surgery; Dermatology and Syphilology; Dextrose-saline; Dilute Strength; Dioptric Strength; Discharge Summary; Disseminated Sclerosis; Dissolved Solids; Donor's Serum; Double Strength; Down's Syndrome; Dry Swallow; Duration of Systole

DSA–Digital Subtraction Angiocardiography; Digital Subtraction Angiography

DSAP–Disseminated Superficial Actinic Porokeratosis

DSAS–Discrete Subaortic Stenosis

DSB–Drug Supervising Body

DSBB–Double Sheath Bronchial Brushing

DSC–Disodium Cromoglycate; Doctor of Surgical Chiropody

DSCG–Disodium Cromoglycate

DSD–Discharge Summary Dictated; Dry Sterile Dressing

DSE–Digital Subtraction Echocardiogram

DSI–Deep Shock Insulin; Digital Subtraction Imaging; Down's Syndrome International

DSIP–Delta Sleep-Inducing Peptide

DSM–Dextrose Solution Mixture; Drink Skim Milk

DSR–Dynamic Spatial Reconstructor

DSS–Dengue Shock Syndrome; Developmental Sentence Scoring; Dioctyl Sodium Sulfosuccinate

DST–Desensitization Test; Dexamethasone Suppression Test; Dihydrostreptomycin; Donorspecific Transfusion

DSUH–Direct Suggestion Under Hypnosis

DSVP–Downstream Venous Pressure

DSX–Detrostix

DT–Delirium Tremens; Dental Technician; Diphtheria and Tetanus; Diphtheria Toxoid; Discharge Tomorrow; Dispensing Tablet; Distance Test; Diversional Therapy; Duration of Tetany

DTBC–Tubocurarine

DTC–Day Treatment Center

DTCD–Diploma in Tuberculosis and Chest Diseases

DTCH–Diploma in Tropical Child Health

DTD–datur talis dosis (give of such a dose)

D-TGA–Dextroposition of the Great Arteries

DTH–Delayed-Type Hypersensitivity

DTLA–Detroit Test of Learning Aptitude

DTMA–Desoxycorticosterone Trimethylacetate

DTMVmax–Diastolic Transmembrane Voltage, Maximum

DTP–Diphtheria, Tetanus and Pertussis; Distal Tingling on Percussion (Tinel's Sign)

DTR–Deep Tendon Reflex

DTS–Dense Tubular System

DTs–Delirium Tremens

DTT–Diphtheria-Tetanus Toxoid; Direct Transverse Traction

DTV–Due to Void

DT-VAC–Diphtheria-tetanus Vaccine

DTX–Detoxification

DTZ–Diatrizoate

DU–Decubitus Ulcer; Density Unknown; Diabetic Urine; Diagnosis Undetermined; Dog Unit; Duodenal Ulcer; Duroxide Uptake

DUB–Dubowitz Score; Dysfunctional Uterine Bleeding

DV–Dianhydrogalactitol and VP-16; Dilute Volume; Distemper Virus; Double Vision

D&V–Diarrhea and Vomiting

DVA–Distance Visual Acuity; Duration of Voluntary Apnea; Vindesine

DVCC–Disease Vector Control Center

DVD–Dissociated Vertical Divergence

DV&D–Diploma in Venereology and Dermatology

DVDALV–Double Vessel Disease with an Abnormal Left Ventricle

DVE–Duck Virus Enteritis

DVI–Digital Vascular Imaging System

DVIU–Direct Vision Internal Urethrotomy

DVLP–Daunomycin, Vincristine, L-asparaginase and Prednisone

DVM–Digital Voltmeter

DVPL-ASP–Daunorubicin, Vincristine, Prednisone and L-asparaginase

DVR–Department of Vocational Rehabilitation; Derotational Varus Osteotomy; Double Valve Replacement

DVT–Deep Vein Thrombosis

DW–Deionized Water; Distilled Water; Dry Weight

DWD–Died with Disease

DWDL–Diffuse, Well-differentiated Lymphoma

DWDLL–Diffuse, Well-differentiated, Lymphocytic Lymphoma

DX–Diagnosis; Diffusing Capacity of the Lung Expressed as Volume

DXM–Dexamethasone

DXR–Deep X-ray; Dextrose

DZ–Disease; Dizziness

DZAPO–Cytosine Arabinoside, Azacytidine, Prednisone, Vincristine and Daunomycin

E

E–Air Dose; Edema; Elastance; Electrode Potential; Emmetropia; Enema; Epinephrine; Erythrocyte; Esophagus; Esophoria; Estradiol; Ethmoid Sinus; Expired; Expired Gas; Eye

E_1–Estrone

E_2–17-beta-Estradiol

E_3–Estriol

E_4–Estetrol

EA–Educational Age; Emergency Area; Endocardiographic Amplifier; Endometriosis Association; Erythrocyte Antibody; Estivoautumnal Malaria; Ethacrynic Acid

EAA–Epilepsy Association of America; Extrinsic Allergic Alveolitis

EAB–Elective Abortion; Ethics Advisory Board

EAC–Ehrlich Ascites Carcinoma; Erythrocyte Antibody Complement; External Auditory Canal

EACA–Epsilon-aminocaproic Acid

EACD–Eczematous Allergic Contact Dermatitis

EAE–Experimental Allergic Encephalomyelitis; Experimental Autoimmune Encephalitis

EAHF–Eczema, Allergy, Hay Fever Complex

EAHLG–Equine Antihuman Lymphoblast Globulin

EAHLS–Equine Antihuman Lymphoblast Serum

EAI–Emphysema Anonymous, Incorporated

EAM–External Auditory Meatus

EAMG–Experimental Autoimmune Myasthenia Gravis

EAN–Experimental Allergic Neuritis

EAP–Electroacupuncture; Employee Assistance Personnel; Epiallopregnanolone

EAST–External Rotation, Abduction, Stress Test

EAT–Ectopic Atrial Tachycardia; Electroaerosol Therapy; Experimental Autoimmune Thymitis

EATC–Ehrlich Ascites Tumor Cell

EB–Elementary Body; Epidermolysis Bullosa; Ebstein-Barr Virus; Estradiol Benzoate

EBAA–Eye Bank Association of America

EBAP–Vindesine, BCNU, Adriamycin and Prednisone

EBD–Epidermolysis Bullosa Dystrophia

EBDD–Epidermolysis Bullosa Dystrophia Dominant

EBF–Erythroblastosis Fetalis

EBI–Electromagnetic Bone Stimulator; Emetine and Bismuth Iodide

EBK–Embryonic Bovine Kidney

EBL–Estimated Blood Loss

EBM–Expressed Breast Milk

EBNA–Epstein-Barr Nuclear Antigen

E/BOD–Electrolyte Biological Oygen Demand

EBS–Electric Brain Stimulator; Emergency Bed Service; Epidermolysis Bullosa Simplex

EC–Ejection Click; Enteric-coated; Entering Complaint; Epidermal Cell; Excitation-contraction; Excitatory Center; Eyes Closed

ECA–Ethacrynic Acid

ECAT–Emission Computerized Axial Tomography

ECBD–Exploration of Common Bile Duct

ECBO–Enteric Cytopathogenic Bovine Orphan

ECBV–Effective Circulating Blood Volume

ECC–Edema, Clubbing and Cyanosis; Electrocorticogram; Emergency Cardiac Care; Endocervical Cone; Endocervical Conization; Endocervical Curettage; Extracorporeal Circulation

ECCE–Extracapsular Cataract Extraction

ECD–Endocardial Cusion Defect

ECDO–Enteric Cytopathic Dog Orphan

ECE–Endocervical Ecchymosis

ECEMG–Evoked Compound Electromyography

ECF–Effective Capillary Flow; Eosinophilic Chemotactic Factor; Extended Care Facility; Extracellular Fluid

ECF-A–Eosinophil Chemotactic Factor of Anaphylaxis

ECFV–Extracellular Fluid Volume

ECG–Echocardiogram; Electrocardiogram

ECGF–Endothelial Cell Growth Factor

ECHO–Enterocytopathogenic Human Orphan Virus; Etoposide, Cyclophosphamide, Adriamycin and Vincristine

ECI–Electrocerebral Inactivity; Extracorporeal Irradiation

ECIB–Extracorporeal Irradiation of the Blood

ECIL–Extracorporeal Irradiation of Lymph

ECL–Extent of Cerebral Lesion; Extracapillary Lesions

ECLT–Euglobulin Clot Lysis Time

ECM–Erythema Chronicum Migrans

E-C Mixture–Ether-Chloroform Mixture

ECMO–Enteric Cytopathic Monkey Orphan Virus; Extracorporeal Membrane Oxygenation

ECMP–Enterocoated Microspheres of Pancrelipase

ECN–Extended Care Nursery

ECoG–Electrocorticogram; Electrocorticography

ECP–Erythrocyte Coproporphyrin; Estradiol Cyclopentanepropionate

ECPO–Enteric Cytopathogenic Porcine Orphan Virus

ECR–Emergency Chemical Restraint

ECRB–Extensor Carpi Radialis Brevis

ECRL–Extensor Carpi Radialis Longus

ECS–Elective Cosmetic Surgery; Electroconvulsive Shock; Extracellular-like Solution

ECSO–Enteric Cytopathic Swine Orphan Virus

ECT–Electroconvulsive Therapy; Emission Computed Tomography; Enteric-Coated Tablet; Euglobulin Clot Test; European Compression Technique

ECU–Extensor Carpi Ulnaris

ECV–Extracellular Volume; Extracorporeal Volume

ED–Effective Dose; Ehlers-Danlos Syndrome; Electrodialysis; Emergency Department;

Entner-Doudoroff Metabolic Pathway; Epidural; Epileptiform Discharge; Erythema Dose; Ethynodiol; Evidence of Disease; Exertional Dyspnea; Extensor Digitorum

EDA–End-Diastolic Area

EDB–Early Dry Breakfast; Ethylene Dibromide; Extensor Digitorum Brevis

EDC–Emergency Decontamination Center; End-Diastolic Counts; Estimated Date of Conception; Estimated Date of Confinement; Extensor Digitorum Communis

EDD–Effective Drug Duration; Enzyme-Digested Delta Endotoxin; Expected Date of Delivery

EDL–End-Diastolic Length; Extensor Digitorum Longus

ED/LD–Emotionally Disturbed/ Learning Disabled

EDM–Early Diastolic Murmur

EDN–Electrodessication

EDNA–Emergency Department Nurses Association

EDP–End-Diastolic Pressure; Epatite Degenerative-Proliferative (Hepatitis Virus)

EDQ–Extensor Digiti Quinti

EDR–Effective Direct Radiation; Electrodermal Response; Electro-dialysis with Reversed Polarity

EDS–Ehlers-Danlos Syndrome

EDTA–Ethylenediaminetetra-acetic Acid

EDU–Eating Disorder Unit

EDV–End-Diastolic Volume

EDVI–End-Diastolic Volume Index

EDW–Estimated Dry Weight

EDWTH–End-Diastolic Wall Thickness

EDXA–Energy-Dispersive X-ray Analysis

EE–Embryo Extract; End-to-End (anastomosis); Equine Encephalitis; Eye to Ear; Erythematous-Edematous

EEA–Electroencephalic Audiometry; End-to-End Anastomosis

EEC–Ectrodactyly, Ectodermal Dysplasia; Enteropathogenic Esche-richia Coli

EEC Syndrome–Ectrodactyly-Ectodermal Dysplasia-Clefting Syndrome

EEE–Eastern Equine Encephalitis; Edema, Erythema and Exudate; Experimental Enterococcal Endocarditis; External Eye Examination

EEEP–End-expiratory Esophageal Pressure

EEG–Electroencephalogram

EEME–Ethinylestradiol Methyl Ether

EENT–Eyes, Ears, Nose and Throat

EEPI–Extraretinal Eye Position Information

EER–Electroencephalic Response

EES–Erythromycin Ethylsuccinate

EF–Ectopic Focus; Edema Factor; Ejection Factor; Ejection Fraction; Embryo-fetal; Emergency Facilities; Emotional Factor; Encephali-togenic Factor; Endurance Factor; Eosinophilic Fasciitis; Equivalent Focus; Extended Field; Extrinsic Factor

EFA–Epilepsy Foundation of America; Essential Fatty Acids; Extrafamily Adoptees

EFAD–Essential Fatty Acid Deficiency

EFE–Endocardial Fibroelastosis
EFM–Electronic Fetal Monitoring
EFVC–Expiratory Flow-Volume Curve
EFW–Estimated Fetal Weight
EG–Esophagogasterctomy; External Genitalia
EGA–Estimated Gestational Age
EGBPS–Equilibrium-Grated Blood Pool Study
EGBUS–External Genitalia and Bartholin's, Urethral and Skene's (Glands)
EGD–Esophagogastroduodenoscopy
EGDF–Embryonic Growth and Development Factor
EGG–Electrogastrogram
EGJ–Esophagogastric Junction
EGL–Eosinophilic Granuloma of the Lung
EGM–Electrogram
EGOT–Erythrocyte Glutamic Oxaloacetic Transaminase
EGS–Electric Galvanic Stimulation
EGTA–Esophagogastric Tube Airway
EH–Educationally Handicapped; Emotionally Handicapped; Enlarged Heart; Essential Hypertension; Extramedullary Hematopoiesis
E&H–Environment and Heredity
EHA–Emotional Health Anonymous
EHAA–Epidermic Hepatitis-Associated Antigen
EHB–Elevate Head of Bed
EHBA–Extrahepatic Biliary Atresia
EHBF–Essential High Blood Pressure; Estimated Hepatic Blood Flow; Exercise Hyperemia Blood Flow
EHC–Enterohepatic Circulation; Enterohepatic Clearance; Essential Hypercholesterolemia; Extended Health Care
EH-CF–Entamoeba Histolytica-Complement Fixation
EHD–Epizootic Hemorrhagic Disease
EHDA–Etidronate Sodium

EHF–Electrohydraulic Fragmentation; Epidemic Hemorrhagic Fever; Exophthalmos-hyperthyroid Factor

EH-IHA–Complement Histolytica-Indirect Hemagglutination

EHL–Effective Half-life; Electrohydraulic Lithotriptor; Endogenous Hyperlipidemia; Extensor Hallucis Longus

EHO–Extrahepatic Obstruction

EHP–Excessive Heat Production; Extrahigh Potency

EHPH–Extrahepatic Portal Hypertension

EHV–Equine Herpes Virus

EI–Electrolyte Imbalance; Eosinophilc Index

E/I–Expiration-Inspiration Ratio

E&I–Endocrine and Infertility

EIA–Electroimmunoassay; Exercise-Induced Anaphylaxis; Exercise-Induced Asthma

EIAB–Extracranial-Intracranial Arterial Bypass

EIB–Exercise-Induced Bronchospasm

EID–Egg-Infective Dose; Electronic Infusion Device

EIDP–Early Intervention Development Profile

EIP–Extensor Indicis Proprius

EIPS–Endogenous Inhibitor of Prostaglandin

EIS–Endoscopic Injection Scleropathy; Epidemic Intelligence Service

EIWA–Escala Inteligencia Wechsler Para Adultes (Wechsler Adult Intelligence Scale)

EJ–Elbow Jerk; External Jugular

EKC–Epidemic Keratoconjunctivitis

EKG–Electrocardiogram

EKY–Electrokymogram

EL–Early Latent; Erythroleukemia; Exercise Limit

E-L–External Lids

ELAT–Enzyme-linked Antiglobulin Test

ELB–Early Light Breakfast

ELF–Elective Low Forceps Delivery

ELH–Endolymphatic Hydrops
ELI–Environmental Language Inventory
ELISA–Enzyme-linked Immunoadsorbent Assay
ELOP–Estimated Length of Program
ELOS–Estimated Length of Stay; Extralymphatic Organ Site
ELP–Endogenous Limbic Potential; Electrophoresis
ELSS–Emergency Life Support System
EM–Ejection Murmur; Emergency Medicine; Emotionally Disturbed; Erythema Multiforme; External Monitor
E-M–Embden-Meyerhof Pathway
E&M–Endocrine and Metabolism
Em–Emmetropia
EMA–Emergency Assistance
EMB–Embryology; Endometrial Biopsy; Endomyocardial Biopsy; Explosive Mental Behavior
EMC–Emergency Medical Care; Encephalomyocarditis; Endometrial Curettage
EMD–Electromechanical Dissociation; Esophageal Motility Disorder
EMF–Emergency Medical Foundation; Endomyocardial Fibrosis; Erythrocyte Maturation Factor; Evaporated Milk Formula
EMG–Electromyelogram; Electromyelography; Essential Monoclonal Gammopathy; Exophthalmos, Macroglossia and Gigantism
EMGORS–Electromyogram Sensors
EMI–Emergency Medical Information
EMIC–Emergency Maternity and Infant Care
EMMA–Eye-movement Measuring Apparatus
EMO–Epstein and Macintosh, Oxford
EMR–Educable Mentally Retarded; Emergency Mechanical Restraint; Empty, Measure and Record
EMS–Electric Muscle Stimulation; Electromyostimulation; Emergency Medical Service
EMT–Emergency Medical Technician; Emergency Medical Treatment

EMV–Eye, Motor and Verbal

EN–Enema; Erythema Nodosum

ENA–Extractable Nuclear Antibodies

ENG–Electronystagmogram

ENL–Erythema Nodosum Leprosum

ENR–Eosinophilic Nonallergic Rhinitis; Extrathyroidal Neck Radioactivity

ENT–Ears, Nose and Throat

ENU–Ethylnitrosurea

EO–Ethylene Oxide; Expected Outcome; Eyes Open

EOA–Esophageal Obturator Airway; Examine, Opinion and Advice

EOG–Electro-Oculogram; Electro-Olfactogram; Ethrane, Oxygen and Gas

EOL–End of Life

EOM–Extraocular Motion; Extraocular Muscle

EOMA–Emergency Oxygen Mask Assembly

EOMF–Extraocular Movements Full

EOMI–Extraocular Motion Intact; Extraocular Muscles Intact

EOR–Exclusive Operating Room

EORA–Elderly Onset Rheumatoid Arthritis

EOS–Ellipse of Skin

EOT–Effective Oxygen Transport

EOU–Epidemic Observation Unit

EOWPVT–Expressive One-Word Picture Vocabulary Test

EP–Ectopic Pregnancy; Edible Portion; Electrophysiologic; Emergency Procedures; Endpoint; Epithelial; Erythrocyte Protoporphyrin; Erythropoietic Porphyria; Esophageal Pressure; Evoked Potential; Extreme Pressure; Protoporphyrin

EPA–Erect Posterior-Anterior

EPB–Environmental Pre-Language Battery; Extensor Pollicis Brevis

EPC–Electronic Pain Control; Epilepsia Partialis Continua; External Pneumatic Compression

EPEC–Enteropathogenic Escherichia Coli

EPEG–Etoposide

EPF–Endothelial Proliferating Factor; Exophthalmos-Producing Factor

EPG–Electropneumogram

EPI–Epithelium; Evoked Potential Index; Eysenck Personality Inventory

EPK–Early Prenatal Karyotype

EPL–Extensor Pollicis Longus

EPLB–Environmental Pre-Language Battery

EPM–Electronic Pacemaker; Energy-Protein Malnutrition

EPP–End-Plate Potential; Equal Pressure Point; Erythropoietic Protoporphyria

EPPS–Edwards Personal Preference Schedule

EPR–Electrophrenic Respiration; Emergency Physical Restraint

EPS–Elastosis Perforans Serpiginosa; Electrophysiologic Study; Exophthalmos-Producing Substance; Extrapyramidal Symptom

EPSP–Excitatory Postsynaptic Potential

EPT–Early Pregnancy Test

EQ–Educational Quotient; Encephalization Quotient

ER–Emergency Room; Ejection Rate; Equivalent Roentgen; Estrogen Receptor; Evoked Response; Extended Release; External Rotation

E&R–Equal and Reactive

ERA–Electrical Response Activity; Electroshock Research Association; Estrogen Receptor Assay; Evoked Response Audiometry

ERBF–Effective Renal Blood Flow

ERC–Endoscopic Retrograde Cholangiography; Enterocytopathogenic Human Orphan Rhinocoryza Virus; Erythropoietin-Responsive Cell

ERCP–Endoscopic Retrograde Cannulation of Pancreatic Duct; Endoscopic Retrograde Cholangiopancreatography

ERD–Evoked Response Detector

ERE–External Rotation in Extension

ERF–External Rotation in Flexion; Eye Research Foundation

ERG–Electroretinogram

ERL–Effective Refractory Length

ERM–Electrochemical Relaxation Methods

ERP–Effective Refractory Period; Endoscopic Retrograde Pancreatography; Equine Rhino-pneumonitis; Estrogen Receptor Protein

ERPF–Effective Renal Plasma Flow

ERSP–Event-Related Slow-Brain Potential

ERT–Estrogen Replacement Therapy

ERV–Expiratory Reserve Volume

ES–Ego Stress; Ejection Sound; Electrical Stimulation; Elopement Status; End-to-Side; Enema Saponis (soap enema); Esophageal Scintigraphy; Endoscopic Sphincterotomy; Exsmoker; Extrasystole; Exterior Surface

ESA–Electrolysis Society of America

ESAP–Evoked Sensory Action Potential

ESB–Electrical Stimulation to Brain

ESC–End-Systolic Counts; Erythropoietin-Sensitive Stem Cells

ESCN–Electrolyte-Produced and Steroid-Produced Cardiopathy Characterized by Necrosis

ESD–Esophagus, Stomach and Duodenum

ESF–Erythropoietic-Stimulating Factor

ESL–End-Systolic Length

ESM–Ejection Systolic Murmur

ESN–Educationally Subnormal; Estrogen-Stimulated Neurophysin

ESO–Electrospinal Orthosis; Esophagus

ESP–Early Systolic Paradox; Effective Sensory Projection; Effective Systolic Pressure; End-Systolic Pressure; Epidermal Soluble Protein; Evoked Synaptic Potential; Extra-sensory Perception

ESR–Electric Skin Resistance; Erythrocyte Sedimentation Rate

ESRD–End-stage Renal Disease

ESS–Erythrocyte-Sensitizing Substance

EST–Electroshock Therapy

ESU–Electrosurgical Unit

ESV–End-Systolic Volume; Esophageal Valve

ESVI–End-systolic Volume Index

ESWL–Extracorporeal Shock Wave Lithotripsy

ET–Ebbinghaus Test; Educational Therapy; Ejection Time; Endotracheal tube; Enterostomal Therapist; Esotropia; Essential Thrombocythemia; Ethionamide; Eustacian Tube; Exercise Treadmill

ETA–Estimated Time of Arrival

ETC–Estimated Time of Conception

ETEC–Enterotoxic Escherichia Coli

ETF–Eustacian Tubal Function

ETM–Erythromycin

ETO–Estimated Time of Ovulation

ETP–Entire Treatment Period; Eustacian Tube Pressure

ETR–Effective Thyroxine Ratio; Epitympanic Recess

ETT–Endotracheal Tube; Exercise Tolerance Test; Extrathyroidal Thyroxine

ETU–Emergency and Trauma Unit; Emergency Treatment Unit

EU–Euthyroid; Excretory Urogram

EUA–Examination Under Anesthesia

EUS–External Urethral Sphincter

EUV–Extreme Ultraviolet Laser

EV–Evoked Response; Extravascular

EVP–Evoked Visual Potential

EVR–Evoked Response

EWB–Estrogen Withdrawal Bleeding

EXBF–Exercise Hyperemia Blood Flow

ExPGN–Extracapillary Proliferative Glomerular Nephritis

EXREM–External Radiation Dose

EX U–Excretory Urogram

EZ–Eczema

F

F–Facial; Farenheit; Feces; Fertility; Field of Vision; Finger; Focal Length; Foramen; Formulary; Fracture; French; Frontal; Frontal Sinus

FA–False Aneurysm; Families Anonymous; Femoral Artery; Fetal Age; Fibrosing Alveolitis; 5-Fluorouracil and Adriamycin; Folic Acid; Forearm; Fortified Aqueous; Freund's Adjuvant; Functional Activities

FAAP–Family Assessment Adjustment Pass

FAB–Antigen-Binding Fragments; Functional Arm Brace

FABER–Flexion in Abduction and External Rotation

FABERE–Flexion, Abduction, External Rotation and Extension

FAC–5-Fluorouracil, Adriamycin and Cyclophosphamide; Fractional Area Concentration

FACA–Fellow of the American College of Anesthetists; Fellow of the American College of Angiology; Fellow of the American College of Apothecaries

FACAL–Fellow of the American College of Allergists

FACAS–Fellow of the American College of Abdominal Surgeons

FAC-BCG–Ftorafur, Adriamycin, Cyclophosphamide and Bacille Calmette-Guerin

FACC–Fellow of the American College of Cardiologists

FACCP–Fellow of the American College of Chest Physicians

FACCPC–Fellow of the American College of Clinical Pharmacology and Chemotherapy

FACD–Fellow of the American College of Dentists

FACFP–Fellow of the American College of Family Physicians

FACFS–Fellow of the American College of Foot Surgeons

FACG–Fellow of the American College of Gastroenterology

FACH–Forceps to After-Coming Head

FACLM–Fellow of the American College of Legal Medicine

FACNP–Fellow of the American College of Neuropsychopharmacology

FACO–Fellow of the American College of Otolaryngology

FACOG–Fellow of the American College of Obstetricians and Gynecologists

FACOS–Fellow of the American College of Orthopedic Surgeons

FACP–Fellow of the American College of Physicians; Ftorafur, Adriamycin, Cyclophosphamide and Cisplatin

FACPM–Fellow of the American College Preventative Medicine

FACR–Fellow of the American College of Radiology

FACS–Fellow of the American College of Surgeons; 5-Fluorouracil, Adriamycin, Cyclophosphamide and Streptozocin

FACSM–Fellow of the American College of Sports Medicine

FACT–Flanagan Aptitude Classification Test

FACVP–5-Fluorouracil, Adriamycin, Cyclophosphamide and VP-16

FAD–Familial Autonomic Dysfunction; Family Assessment Device; Fetal Activity-Acceleration Determination

FADIR–Flexion in Adduction and Internal Rotation

FAI–Functional Assessment Inventory

FAM–5-Fluorouracil, Adriamycin and Mitomycin-C

FAM-C–5-Fluorouracil, Adriamycin and Mitomycin-C

FAME–5-Fluorouracil, Adriamycin and Methyl-CCNU

FANA–Fluorescent Antinuclear Antibody

F and R–Force and Rhythm

FANPT–Freeman Anxiety Neurosis and Psychosomatic Test

FANS–Fellow of the American Neurological Society

FAP–Familial Amyloid Polyneuropathy; Fibrillating Action Potentials; 5-Fluorouracil, Adriamycin and Cisplatin

FAPA–Fellow of the American Psychiatric Association

FAS–Fetal Alcohol Syndrome

FASC–Free-standing Ambulatory Surgical Center

FAST–Flow-Assisted, Short-Term Ballon Catheter; Fluorescent Allergosorbent Test

FAT–Fluorescent Antibody Technique; Food Awareness Training

FB–Fasting Blood Sugar; Feedback; Fiberoptic Bronchoscopy; Foreign Body

FBCOD–Foreign Body of Cornea, Oculus Dexter

FBCOS–Foreign Body of Cornea, Oculus Sinister

FBD–Functional Bowel Disorder

FBF–Forearm Blood Flow

FBG–Fibrinogen

FBH–Familial Benign Hypocalciuric Hypercalcemia

FBI–Flossing, Brushing and Irrigation

FBL–Follicular Basal Lamina

FBP–Femoral Blood Pressure; Fibrinogen Breakdown Products

FBRCM–Fingerbreadth Below Right Costal Margin

FBS–Fasting Blood Sugar; Feedback Signal

FBU–Fingers Below Umbilicus

FC–Fever and Chills; Finger Clubbing; Finger Counting; Foley Catheter; Functional Class

F&C–Flare and Cells; Foam and Condom

5-FC–5-Fluorocytosine

Fc–Crystallizable Fragment

FCA–Freund's Complete Adjuvant

FCAP–Fellow of the College of American Pathologists

FCC–Familial Colonic Cancer; Fracture, Compound and Comminuted

FCCP–Fellow of the American College of Chest Physicians

FCD–Fecal Collection Device

FCDB–Fibrocystic Disease of the Breast

FCG–French Catheter Gauge

FCH–Familial Combined Hyperlipidemia

FChS–Fellow of the Society of Chiropodists

FCMC–Family-Centered Maternity Care

FCMD–Fukiyama's Congenital Muscular Dystrophy
FCMN–Family-centered Maternity Nursing
FCMS–Fellow of the College of Medicine and Surgery
FCMW–Foundation for Child Mental Welfare
FCO–Fellow of the College of Osteopathy
FCP–Final Common Pathway
FCR–Flexor Carpi Radialis; Fractional Catabolic Rate
FCRA–Fecal Collection Receptacle Assembly
FCRB–Flexor Carpi Radialis Brevis
FCS–Fecal Containment System; Feedback Control System
FCSNVD–Fever, Chills, Sweating, Nausea, Vomiting and Diarrhea
FCST–Fellow of the Chartered Society of Physiotherapy
FCT–Food Composition Table
FCU–Flexor Carpi Ulnaris
FD–Familial Dysautonomia; Fan Douche; Fatal Dose; Focal Distance;
    Foot Drape; Forceps Delivery
F&D–Fixed and Dilated
FDA–Frenchay Dysarthria Assessment; Frontodextra Anterior
FDE–Final Drug Evaluation
FDF–Fast Death Factor
FDIU–Fetal Death in Utero
FDL–Flexor Digitorum Longus
FDLMP–First Day of Last Menstrual Period
FDP–Fibrin Degradation Products; Flexor Digitorum Profundus;
    Flexor Distal Phalanx;
Frontodextra Posterior
FDQB–Flexor Digiti Quinti Brevis
FDS–Fellow in Dental Surgery; Flexor Digitorum Sublimis; Flexor
    Digitorum Superficialis; For Duration of Stay
FDT–Frontodextra Transversa
FDTVMP–Frostig Developmental Test of Visual-Motor Perception
FE–Fecal Emesis; Fecal Energy; Fetal Erythroblastosis; Fluid Extract

Fe–Female; Iron (chemical symbol)

FEBP–Fetoneonatal Estrogen-Binding Protein

FEC–Fecal; Forced Expiratory Capacity; Free Erythrocyte Coproporphyrin

FECG–Fetal Electrocardiogram

FECP–Free Erythrocyte Coproporphyria

FECT–Fibroelastic Connective Tissue

FECV–Functional Extracellular Fluid Volume

FEE–Forced Equilibrilating Expiration

FEF–Forced Expiratory Flow

FEKG–Fetal Electrocardiogram

FEL–Familial Erythrophagocytic Lymphohistiocytosis

FEMED–5-Fluorouracil, Methotrexate, Cyclophosphamide and Prednisone

FEOM–Full Extraocular Motion

FEP–Free Erythrocyte Protoporphyrin

FES–Forced Expiratory Spirogram

FET–Fixed Erythrocyte Turnover; Forced Expiratory Time

FETS–Forced Expiratory Time in Seconds

FEUO–For External Use Only

FEV–Forced Expiratory Volume

FF–Fat-free; Fecal Frequency; Fertility Factor; Finger-to-Finger; Flat Feet; Flip-Flop; Force Fluids; Forearm Flow; Fundus Firm; Further Flexion

F&F–Filiform and Follower

FFA–Free Fatty Acids; Fellow of the Faculty of Anesthetists

FFC–Fixed Flexion Contracture

FFD–Fellow in the Faculty of Dentistry; Focus Film Distance

FFI–Free From Infection

FFP–Fresh Frozen Plasma; Fistful of Prisms

FFR–Fellow of the Faculty of Radiologists

FFS–Fat-free Solids; Fat-Free Supper

FFT–Fast-Fourier Transforms; Flicker Fusion Threshold

FFU–Focus-Forming Unit

FGD–Fatal Granulomatous Disease

FGLU–Fasting Glucose

FGS–Focal Glomerulosclerosis

FH–Familial Hypercholesteremia; Family History; Fetal head; Fetal Heart; Frankfort Horizontal Plane of Skull; Fundal Height

FHF–Fulminate Hepatic Failure

FHH–Familial Hypocalciuric Hypercalcemia; Fetal Heart Heard

FHI–Fuch's Heterochromic Iridocyclitis

FHNH–Fetal Heart not Heard

FHR–Familial Hypophosphatemic Rickets; Fetal Heart Rate

FHS–Fetal Heart Sounds; Fetal Hydantoin Syndrome

FHT–Fetal Heart Tone

FHVP–Free Hepatic Vein Pressure

FI–Fever Caused by Infection; Fixed Internal; Forced Inspiration

FIA–Freund's Incomplete Adjuvant

FIB–Fibrositis; Fibrinogen; Fibrillation; Fibula

FIC–Fasting Intestinal Contents

FICO2–Fraction of Inspired Carbon Dioxide

FICU–Fetal Intensive Care Unit

FID–Free Induction Decay or Delay

FIF–Feedback Inhibition Factor; Fibroblast Interferon; Forced Inspiratory Flow

FIFR–Fasting Intestinal Flow Rate

FIGO–International Federation of Gynecology and Obstetrics

FIH–Fat-induced Hyperglycemia

FIME–5-Fluorouracil, ICRF-159 and Methyl-CCNU

FIN–Fine Intestinal Needle

F-Insulin–Fibrous Insulin

FIO2–Forced Inspiratory Oxygen; Fractional Concentration of Inspired Oxygen; Inspired Flow of Oxygen

FIRDA–Frontal Intermittent Rhythmic Delta Activity

FIT–Fusion Inferred Threshold Test

FITT–Frequency, Intensity, Time and Type

FIUO–For Internal Use Only

FIVC–Forced Inspiratory Vital Capacity

FJN–Familial Juvenile Nephrophthisis

FJRM–Full Joint Range of Motion

FL–Fluid; Focal Length; Frontal Lobe

FLA–Frontolaeva Anterior (Left Frontoanterior Fetal Position)

FLC–Friend Leukemia Cells

FLK–Funny-Looking Kid

FLP–Few Large Platelets; Frontolaeva Posterior (Left Frontoposterior Fetal Position)

FLS–Fibrous Long-Spacing Collagen; Flashing Lights and/ or Scotoma

FLSA–Follicular Lymphosarcoma

FLSP–Fluorescein-Labeled Serum Protein

FLT–Frontolaeva Transversa (Left Frontotransverse Fetal Position)

FLTA–Fullerton Language Test for Adolescents

FLTAC–Fisher-Logemann Test of Articular Competence

FLV–Friend Leukemia Virus

FM–Face Mask; Farnsworth-Munsell; Feedback Mechanism; Fetal Movements; Forensic Medicine; Formerly Married; Foster Mother; Frequency Modulation

F.M.–Fiat Mistura (Make a Mixture)

F&M–Firm and Midline

FMB–Full Maternal Behavior

FMC–Fetal Movement Count

FMCA–Forensic Medicine Consultant Advisor

FMD–Fibromuscular Dysplasia; Foot-and-Mouth Disease

FME–Full Mouth Extraction

FMF–Familial Mediterranean Fever; Fetal Movement Felt; Forced Midexpiratory Flow

FMG–Fine Mesh Gauze
FMH–Fat-Mobilizing Hormone; Fibromuscular Hyperplasia
FMIV–Forced Mandatory Intermittent Ventilation
FMP–Fasting Metabolic Panel; First Menstrual Period
FMS–Full Mouth Series
FMX–Full Mouth Radiography
FN–False Negative; Finger-to-Nose
FNA–Fine Needle Aspiration
FNAB–Fine Needle Aspiration Biopsy
FNCJ–Fine Needle Catheter Jejunostomy
FNF–Finger-Nose-Finger Test
FNH–Focal Nodular Hyperplasia
FNP–Family Nurse Practitioner
FNR–False Negative Rate
FNS–Functional Neuromuscular Stimulation
FO–Fiberoptic; Foramen Ovale; Fronto-Occipital
FOA–Federation of Orthodontic Associations
FOAVF–Failure of all Vital Forces
FOB–Father of Baby; Fecal Occult Blood; Feet Out of Bed; Fiberoptic
   Bronchoscopy
FOC–Father of Child
FOD–Free of Disease
FOG–Fluothane, Oxygen and Gas
FOI–Flight of Ideas
FOM–5-Fluorouracil, Oncovin and Mitomycin-C
FOOB–Fell Out of Bed
FOPR–Full Outpatient Rate
FOVI–Field of Vision Intact
FP–False Positive; Family Planning; Family Practitioner; Flat Plate;
   Fluid Pressure; Food Poisoning; Frontoparietal; Frozen Plasma;
   Fundal Pressure
F-P–Femoral-Popliteal

FPA–Family Planning Association

FPAL–Full-Term Deliveries, Premature Deliveries, Abortions and Living Children

FPB–Femoral-Popliteal Bypass; Flexor Pollicis Brevis

FPC–Family Planning Clinic; Fish Protein Concentrate

FPD–Fetopelvic Disproportion; Fixed Partial Denture

FPDVP–Frostig Program for the Development of Visual Perception

FPG–Fasting Plasma Glucose

FPHE–Formalin-Treated Pyruvaldehyde-Stabilizing Human Erythrocytes

FPL–Flexor Pollicis Longus

FPNA–First-pass Nuclear Angiocardiography

FPRA–First-pass Radionuclide Angiogram

FPS–Fellow of the Pathological Society; Fellow of the Pharmaceutical Society

FPSLST–Fluharty Preschool Speech and Language Screening test

FPT–Fixed Parenchymal Turnover

FPVB–Femoral-Popliteal Vein Bypass

FPZ–Fluphenazine

FR–Failure Rate; Fibrinogen-Related; Flow Rate

F&R–Force and Rhythm

Fr–French; Franklin

FRA–Fluorescent Rabies Antibody

FRC–Federal Radiation Council; Functional Residual Capacity; Frozen Red Cells

FRF–Fertility Research Foundation; Follicle-Stimulating Hormone-Releasing Factor

FRJM–Full Range of Joint Movement

FRP–Functional Refractory Period

FRS–Furosemide; Ferredoxin-Reducing Substance

FRT–Family Relations Test; Full Recovery Time

FS–Factor of Safety; Flexible Sigmoidoscopy; Forearm Supinated; Fracture, Simple; Frozen Section; Full and Soft; Full-Scale Intelligence Quotient

FSB–Fetal Scalp Blood; Fokes Sentence Builder

FSBM–Full-Strength Breast Milk

FSBT–Fowler Single Breath Test

FSC–Forer Sentence Completion Test; Fracture, Simple, Comminuted

FSD–Focal Skin Distance

FSE–Fetal Scalp Electrode

FSF–Fibrin Stabilizing Factor

FSG–Focal and Segmental Glomerulosclerosis

FSH–Facioscapulohumeral; Follicle-Stimulating Hormone

FSHMD–Facioscapulohumeral Muscular Dystrophy

FSHRF–Follicle-stimulating Hormone Releasing Factor

FSIA–Foot Shock-Induced Analgesia

FSP–Fibrin Split Products

FSR–Fellow of the Society of Radiographers; Fusiform Skin Revision

FSR-3–Isoniazid

FSS–French Steel Sound Dilator

FST–Foam Stability Test

FSU–Family Service Unit

FT–False Transmitter; Family Therapy; Fibrous Tissue; Follow Through; Fourier Transform; Free Thyroxine; Full Term; Functional Test

FTBD–Fit to be Detained; Full-Term Born Dead

FTD–Failure to Descend; Femoral Total Density

FTF–Finger-to-Finger; Free Thyroxine Fraction

FTG–Full Thickness Graft

FTI–Free Thyroxine Index

FTLB–Full-Term Living Birth

FTLFC–Full-Term Living Female Child

FTLMC–Full-Term Living Male Child

FTM–Fractional Test Meal

FTN–Finger-to-Nose; Full-Term Nursery
FTND–Full-Term Normal Delivery
FTP–Failure to Progress
FTR–For the Record
FTSG–Full Thickness Skin Graft
FTT–Failure to Thrive; Fixed Tissue Turnover
FU–Fecal Urobilinogen; Fluorouracil; Follow-up; Fractional Urinalysis
F&U–Flanks and Upper Quadrants
5FU–5-Fluorouracil
FUB–Functional Uterine Bleeding
FUDR–Floxuridine
FUE–Fever of Undetermined Etiology
FUM–5-Fluorouracil and Methotrexate
FUN–Follow-up Note
FUO–Fever of Undetermined Origin; Fever of Unknown Origin
FUR–Fluorouracil Riboside
FURAM–Ftorafur, Adriamycin and Mitomycin-C
F-V–Flow Volume
FVC–Forced Vital Capacity
FVH–Focal Vascular Headache
FVL–Femoral Vein Ligation; Flow Volume Loop
FVR–Forearm Vascular Resistance
FW–Felix-Weil; Forced Whisper; Fragment Wound
FWA–Family Welfare Association
FWB–Full Weight Bearing
FWHM–Full-Width Half-Maximum
FXN–Function
FXR–Fracture
FYA–Duffy A Positive
FYAN–Duffy A Negative
FYB–Duffy B Positive
FYBN–Duffy B Negative

FYI–For Your Information
FZ–Focal Zone
FZRC–Frozen Red Blood Cells

G

G–Conductance; Gallop; Gas; Gingival; Glucose; Glycine; Grafenberg
  Spot; Gravida; Gross
g–Gender; Gravida
GA–Gastric Analysis; General Anesthesia; General Appearance;
  Gestational Age; Gingivoaxial; Gramicidin A; Gut-Associated
Ga–Airway Conductance; Gallium; Granulocyte Agglutination
GABA–Gamma-Aminobutyric Acid
GABHS–Group A Beta-Hemolytic Streptococcus
GADS–Gonococcal Arthritis/Dermatitis Syndrome
GAG–Glycosaminoglycan
GALT–Gut-Associated Lymphoid Tissue
GAP–Group for the Advancement of Psychiatry
GAS–Gastroenterology; General Adaptation Syndrome; Generalized
  Arteriosclerosis; Global Assessment Score
GAT–Group Adjustment Therapy
GAW–Airway Conductance
GB–Gallbladder; Guillain-Barre
GBA–Ganglionic-Blocking Agent; Gingivobuccoaxial
GBBHS–Group B Beta-Hemolytic Streptococcus
GBD–Gallbladder Disease
GBG–Gonadal Steroid-Binding Globulin
GBL–Glomerular Basal Lamina
GBP–Gastric Bypass
GBS–Gallbladder Series; Glycerine-Buffered Saline; Group B Beta-
  Hemolytic Streptococcus; Guillain-Barre Syndrome

GBSS–Grey's Balanced Salt Solution

GC–Ganglion Cells; Geriatric Care; Geriatric Chair; Glucocorticoid; Granular Cysts

Gc–Gonococcus

GCA–Giant Cell Arteritis

GCDFP–Gross Cystic Disease Fluid Protein

GCFT–Gonorrhea Complement-Fixation Test

GCIIS–Glucose Control Insulin Infusion System

GC-MS–Gas Chromatography-Mass Spectrometry

GCN–Giant Cerebral Neuron

GCS–Glascow Coma Scale

GCT–Giant Cell Tumor

GD–Gonadal Dysgenesis; Grave's Disease

G&D–Growth and Development

GDD–Gay Disaster Disease (AIDS)

GDM–Gestational Diabetes Mellitus

GDS–Gesell Developmental Schedules; Gradual Dosage Schedule

GE–Gastroemotional; Gastroenteritis; Gastroesophageal; Gastroenterostomy; Gentamicin; Gel Electrophoresis

Ge–Germanium (Chemical symbol)

GEJ–Gastroesophageal Junction

GEMS–Good Emergency Mother Substitute

GEP–Gastroenteropancreatic

GER–Gastroesophageal Reflux

GERL–Golgi-Associated Endoplasmic Reticulum Lysosomes

GES–Glucose Electrolyte Solution

GET–Gastric Emptying Time

GF–Gastric Fistula; Gastric Fluid; Glomerular Filtrate; Gluten-Free; Growth Factor

GFD–Gluten-Free Diet; Goodenough Figure Drawing

GFR–Glomerular Filtration Rate

GFTA–Goldman-Fristoe Test of Articulation

GG–Gamma-Globulin; Guaifenesin
GGA–General Gonadotropic Activity
GGE–General Gland Enlargement
GH–Glenohumeral; Growth Hormone
GHD–Growth Hormone Deficiency
GHDT–Goodenough-Harris Drawing Test
GHQ–General Health Questionnaire
GHRF–Growth Hormone Releasing Factor
GHRH–Growth Hormone Releasing Hormone
GI–Gastroenterology; Gastrointestinal; Globulin Insulin; Granuloma
    Inguinale; Growth-Inhibiting; Gravida I
GIA–Gastrointestinal Anastomosis
GIB–Gastric Ileal Bypass
GIC–General Immunocompetence
GIF–Growth Hormone Inhibiting Factor
GIFT–Gamete Intrafallopian Transfer
GIH–Gastrointestinal Hormone; Growth-Inhibiting Hormone
GII–Gastrointestinal Infection
GIK–Glucose, Insulin and Potassium
GIP–Gastric Inhibitory Peptide; Giant Cell Interstitial Pneumonia
GIS–Gas in Stomach; Gastrointestinal Series; Gastrointestinal System
GIT–Gastrointestinal Tract
GITS–Gastrointestinal Therapeutic System
GITSG–Gastrointestinal Tumor Study Group
GITT–Glucose-Insulin Tolerance Test
GJ–Gap Junctions; Gastrojejunostomy
GKMDT–Graham-Kendall Memory for Designs Test
GL–Greatest Length
GLA–Gingivolinguoaxial
GLI–Glicentin; Glucagon-Like Immunoreactivity
GL-PP–Postprandial Glucose
Gltn–Glomerulotubulonephritis

GM–Gastric Mucosa; Grand Mal Seizure; General Medicine; Grand Multiparity; Monosialoganglioside

GMP–Guanosine Monophosphate

GN–Glomerulonephritis

GNBM–Gram-Negative Bacillary Meningitis

GNID–Gram-Negative Intracellular Diplococci

GNP–Gerontological Nurse Practitioner

GnRF–Gonadotropin-Releasing Factor

G&O–Gas and Oxygen

GOE–Gas, Oxygen and Ether

GOG–Gynecological Oncology Group

GOR–General Operating Room

GORT–Gilmore Oral Reading Test; Gray Oral Reading Test

GOT–Aspartate Aminotransferase; Glutamic-Oxaloacetic Transaminase

GP–General Paralysis; General Paresis; General Practice; Genetic Prediabetes; Globus Pallidus; Goodpasture Syndrome; Gram-Positive; Gutta-Percha

GPA–Gravida, Para and Abortus; Group Practice Association

GPB–Glossopharyngeal Breathing

GPC–Gastric Parietal cell; Giant Papillary Conjunctivitis

GPF–Granulocytosis-Promoting Factor

GPI–General Paralysis of the Insane; Glucose, Potassium and Insulin

Gply–Gingivoplasty

GPM–General Preventative Medicine

GPMAL–Gravida, Para, Multiple Births, Abortions and Live Births

GPPQ–General Purpose Psychiatric Questionnaire

GPT–Glutamate Pyruvate Transaminase

GPUT–Galactose Phosphate Uridyl Transferase

GR–Gamma Ray; Gastric Resection; General Research

GRAE–Generally Regarded as Effective

GRAS–Generally Recognized as Safe

GRD–Gastroesophageal Reflux

GRF–Gonadotropin-Releasing Factor

GRH–Growth Hormone Releasing Hormone

GRPS–Glucose-Ringer-Phosphate Solution

GS–Gastric Shield; General Surgery; Gilbert's Syndrome; Glomerular Sclerosis

GSA–General Somatic Afferent; Gross virus Antigen

GSBG–Gonadal Steroid-Binding Globulin

GSC–Gas-Solid Chromatography; Glascow Scale

GSCN–Giant Serotonin-Containing Neuron

GSD–Genetically Significant Dose

GSE–General Somatic Efferent; Glutagen-Sensitive Enteropathy; Grip Strong and Equal

GSF–Galactosemic Fibroblasts

GSH–Glomerular-Stimulating Hormone; Growth-Stimulating Hormone; Reduced Glutathione

GSI–Genuine Stress Incontinence

GSP–Galvanic Skin Potential

GSPN–Greater Superficial Petrosal Neurectomy

GSR–Galvanic Skin Reflex; Galvanic Skin Response; Generalized Shwartzman Reaction

GST–Graphic Stress Telethermometry

GT–Gait Training; Gastrostomy; Gastrotomy Tube; Gingiva Treatment; Glucose Tolerance; Greater Trochanter; Group Therapy

G&T–Gowns and Towels

GTD–Gestational Trophoblastic Disease

GTF–Glucose Tolerance Factor

GTH–Gonadotropic Hormone

GTN–Gestational Trophoblastic Neoplasia; Glomerulotubulonephritis

GTO–Golgi Tendon Organ

GTT–Glucose Tolerance Test; Guttae (Drops)

GU–Gastric Ulcer; Genitourinary; Glycogenic Unit; Gonococcal Urethritis; Gravitational Ulcer

GUS–Genitourinary Sphincter; Genitourinary System

GV–Gentian Violet; Gingivectomy; Gross Virus

GVA–General Visceral Afferent

GVE–General Visceral Efferent

GVF–Good Visual Fields

GVH–Graft Versus Host

GVHD–Graft Versus Host Disease

GVHR–Graft Versus Host Reaction

Gvty–Gingivectomy

GW–Glycerine in Water

GXD–Graded

GXD EKG–Graded Exercise Electrocardiogram

GXT–Graded Exercise Test

Gy–Gray

GYN–Gynecology

GZ–Guilford-Zimmerman Personality Test

H

H–Head; Heart; Heelstick; Hemisphere; Heparin; Heroin; Homosexual; Hormone; Hour; Hydrogen (Chemical symbol); Hypermetropia; Hyperphoria; Hyperplasia; Hypothalamus; Hypodermic; Vectorcardiogram Electrode (At Neck)

HA–Hallux Abductus; Headache; Hearing Aid; Height Age; Hemolytic Anemia; Hepatic Artery; Hepatitis A; Hepatitis-Associated; Heyden Antibiotic; High Anxiety; Hounsfield; Hyperalimentation; Hypothalamic Amenorrhea

Ha–Absolute Hypermetropia; Hahnium (Chemical symbol)

HAA–Hearing Aid Amplifier; Hemolytic Anemia Antigen; Hepatitis-Associated Antigen

HAB–Hepatitis B

HABF–Hepatic Artery Blood Flow

HAC–Hexamethylmelamine, Adriamycin and Cyclophosphamide

HACS–Hyperactive Child Syndrome

HAD–Hearing Aid Dispenser; Hexamethylmelamine, Adriamycin and Cisplatin

HADD–Hydroxyapatite Deposition Disease

HAE–Hearing Aid Evaluation; Hepatic Embolization; Hereditary Angioedema

HAAg–Hepatitis A Antigen

HAI–Hemagglutination Inhibition; Hepatic Arterial Infusion

HAL–Hyperalimentation

HAM–Hearing Aid Microphone; Hexamethylmelamine, Adriamycin and L-phenylalanine Mustard

HAM-A–Hamilton Anxiety Scale

HAM-D–Hamilton Depression Scale

HAM-II–Hexamethylmelamine, Adriamycin and Methotrexate

HAMP–Hexamethylmelamine, Adriamycin, Methotrexate and Cisplatin

HAN–Heroin-Associated Nephropathy; Hyperplastic Alveolar Nodules

H and P–History and Physical

H and V–Hemigastrectomy and Vagotomy

HANE–Hereditary Angioneurotic Edema

HAO–Hearing Aid Follow-Up and Orientation

HAP–Heredopathia Atactica Polyneuritiformis; Handicapped Aid Program

HAPC–Hospital-Acquired Penetration Contact

HAPE–High-Altitude Pulmonary Edema

HAPS–Hepatic Arterial Perfusion Scintigraphy

HAQ–Headache Assessment Questionnaire

HAS–Highest Asymptomatic Dose; Hyperalimentation Solution; Hypertensive Arteriosclerosis

HASCVD–Hypertensive Arteriosclerotic Cardiovascular Disease

HASP–Hospital Admission and Surveillance Program

HAT–Harmonic Attenuation Table; Head, Arms and Trunk

HATH–Heterosexual Attitudes Towards Homosexuality

HAV–Hallux Abducto Valgus; Hepatitis A Virus

HB–Bundle of His; Heart Block; Hemoglobin; Hepatitis B; Hold Breakfast; House-Bound

Hb-Hemoglobin

HBB–Hospital Blood Bank

Hb CS–Hemoglobin Constant Spring

HBD–Has Been Drinking

HBE–His Bundle Electrogram

HBF–Hand Blood Flow

HBGM–Home Blood Glucose Monitoring

HBHC–Home-Based Hospital Care

HBI–Hemibody Irridiation; High-Serum-Bound Iron

HBIG–Hepatitis B Immunoglobulin

HBLLSB–Heard Best at Left Lower Sternal Border

HBLUSB–Heard Best at Left Upper Sternal Border

HBLV–Human B-Lymphotropic Virus

HBO–Hyperbaric Oxygen

HBP–High Blood Pressure

HBS–Health Behavior Scale; Hemoglobin S

HBSS–Hank's Balanced Salt Solution

HBT–Human Breast Tumor

HBV–Hepatitis B Vaccine; Hepatitis B Virus

HBW–High Birth Weight

HC–Handicapped; Head Circumference; Heart Cycle; Hickman Catheter; Hippocampus; Huntington's Chorea; Hydrocortisone

HCA–Health Care Aide; Heart Cell Aggregate; Hepatocellular Adenoma; Hydrocortisone Acetate

HCAP–Hexamethylmelamine, Adriamycin, Cyclophosphamide and Cisplatin

HCC–Hepatitis Contagiosa Canis; Hepatocellular Carcinoma; Hydroxycholecalciferol

HCD–Heavy Chain Disease; Homologous Canine Distemper

HCF–High Carbohydrate, High Fiber

HCG–Human Chorionic Gonadotropin

HCGN–Hypocomplementemic Glomerulonephritis

Hclmp–Hydrocolloid Impression

HCL–Hairy Cell Leukemia; Hard Contact Lens

HCLF–High Carbohydrate, Low Fiber

HCM–Hypertrophic Cardiomyopathy

HCO_3–Bicarbonate

HCP–Handicapped; Hepatocatalase Peroxidase; Hereditary Coproporphyria

H&CP–Hospital and Community Psychiatry

HCR–Hysterical Conversion Reaction

HCS–Hourglass Contraction of Stomach; Human Chorionic Somatomammotropin; Human Cord Serum

HCT–Heart-Circulation Training; Hematocrit; Human Chorionic Placental Thyrotropin; Hydrochlorothiazide; Hydrocortisone

HCTU–Home Cervical Traction unit

HCU–Homocystinuria

HCVD–Hypertensive Cardiovascular Disease

HD–Hansen's Disease; Hearing Distance; Heart Disease; Heloma Durum (Hard Corn); Hemodialysis; Herniated Disc; High Dosage; High Dose; Hip Disarticulation; Hodgkin's Disease; Huntington's Disease; Hydatid Disease

HDA–Huntington's Disease Association; Hydroxydopamine

HDCCAMS–High-Dose Cyclophosphamide and Adriamycin

HDCV–Human Diploid Cell Rabies Vaccine

HDD–Higher Dental Diploma

HDFP–Hypertension Detection and Follow-Up Program

HDH–Heart Disease History

HDL–High-Density Lipoprotein

HDLW–Distance at Which a Watch is Heard by the Left Ear

HDMTX–High-Dose Methotrexate

HDN–Hemolytic Disease of the Newborn; High-Density Nebulizer

HDPAA–Heparin-Dependent Platelet-Associated Antibody

HDRF–Heart Disease Research Foundation

HDRS–Hamilton Depression Rate Scale

HDRV–Human Diploid Cell Strain Rabies Vaccine

HDRW–Distance at Which a Watch is Heard by the Right Ear

HDS–Herniated Disc Syndrome; Hospital Discharge Survey

HDU–Hemodialysis Unit

HE–Hard Exudate; Hemagglutinating Encephalomyelitis; Hemoglobin Electrophoresis; Hepatic Encephalopathy; Hereditary Elliptocytosis; Human Enteric Virus; Hypogonadotropic Eunuchoidism; Hypophysectomy

H&E–Hemorrhage and Exudate; Heredity and Environment; Hematoxylin and Eosin

H-E–Heat Exchanger

He–Helium (Chemical symbol)

HEA–Human Erythrocyte Antigen

HEART–Health Evaluation and Risk Tabulation

HEB–Hematoencephalic Barrier

HEC–Health Evaluation Center

HEENT–Head, Ears, Eyes, Nose and Throat

HEE Syndrome–Hemiconvulsion, Hemiplegia and Epilepsy Syndrome

HEG–Hemmorhagic Erosive Gastritis

HEHR–Highest Equivalent Heart Rate

HEIR–Health Effects of Ionizing Radiation; High-Energy Ionizing Radiation

HEIS–High-Energy Ion Scattering

HEL–Human Erythroleukemia

HELLP–Hemolysis, Elevated Liver Enzymes and Low Platelets

HELP–Health Emergency Loan Program; Heat Escape Lessening Posture; Henry's Emergency Lessons for People Heroin Emergency Life Project

HEMA–Hematology Profile

HEMPAS–Hereditary Rrythroblastic Multinuclearity with a Positive Acidified Serum Test

HEN–Hemorrhages, Exudates and/or Nicking

HEP–Hepatic; Histamine Equivalent Prick

HEPA–High-Efficiency Particulate Air

HEP-AC–Hepatitis Battery-Acute

HES–Hypereosinophilic Syndrome

HET–Helium Equilibration Time

HEXA-CAF–Hexamethylmelamine, Cyclophosphamide, 5-Fluorouracil and Methotrexate

HEXL–Methohexital

HF–Hageman Factor; Hard-Filled Capsules; Hay Fever; Heart Failure; Hemorrhagic Factor; Hemorrhagic Fever; High Fat; High Flow; High Frequency; Hollow Fiber; House Formula

HFC–Hand-Filled Capsules; Hard-Filled Capsules

HFD–High Forceps Delivery

HFHL–High-Frequency Hearing Loss

HFI–Hereditary Fructose Intolerance

HFJV–High-Frequency Jet Ventilation

HFO–High-Frequency Oscillation

HFOV–High-Frequency Oscillatory Ventilation

HFPPV–High-Frequency Positive Pressure Ventilation

HFRS–Hemorrhagic Fever with Renal Syndrome

HFSH–Human Follicle-Stimulating Hormone

HG–Hemoglobin; Herpes Genitalis; Human Gonadotropin; Human Growth Factor

HGB EL–Hemoglobin Electrophoresis

HGB-PL–Hemoglobin Plasma

HGBS–Methemoglobin-Sulfhemoglobin

HGF–Hyperglycemic-Glycogenolytic Factor

HGG–Human Gamma Globulin

HGH–Human Growth Hormone

HGO–Hepatic Glucose Output

HH–Hard of Hearing; Henderson and Haggard Inhaler; Hiatal Hernia; Hypogonadism; Hypo-gonadotrophic

H&H–Hemoglobin and Hematocrit

HHA–Hereditary Hemolytic Anemia; Home Health Agency; Hypothalamic-Hypophyseal-Adrenal

HHC–Home Health Care

HHD–Hypertensive Heart Disease

HHFM–High-Humidity Face Mask

HHHO–Hypotonia-Hypomentia-Hypogonadism-Obesity

HHN–Hand-Held Nebulizer

HHNK–Hyperglycemic, Hyperosmolar, Nonketotic Coma

HHT–Hereditary Hemorrhagic Telangiectasia

HI–Head Injury; Hemagglutination Inhibition Titer; Hepatobiliary Imaging; High Impulsiveness; Homicidal Ideation

HIB–Hemophilus Influenzae, Type B

HIC–Heart Information Center

HID–Headache, Insomnia and Depression Syndrome

HIDA–Hepatoiminodiacetic Acid

HIE–Hypoxic-Ischemic Encephalopathy

HIF–Higher Integrative Functions

HIHA–High Impulsiveness, High Anxiety

HIL–Hypoxic-Ischemic Lesion

HILA–High Impulsiveness, Low Anxiety

HIO–Hypoiodidism

HIR–Head Injury Routine

HIS–Hospital Information Systems; Health Interview Survey; Health Information Service

HIT–Hemagglutination-Inhibition Test; Heparin Induced Thrombocytopenia; Histamine Inhalation Test; Hypertrophic Infiltrative Tendinitis

HIV–Human Immunodeficiency Virus

HIVD–Herniated Intervertebral Disc

HJ–Hepatojugular; Howell-Jolly Bodies

HJR–Hepatojugular Reflex

HK–Heat-Killed; Heal-to-Knee

HKAFO–Hip-Knee-Ankle-Foot Orthosis

HKLM–Heat-Killed Listeria Monocytogenes

HKO–Hip-Knee Orthosis

HKS–Heel-Knee-Shin Test

HL–Haalux Limitus; Haloperidol; Hairline; Harelip; Hearing Level; Hearing Loss; Heparin Lock; Hickman Line; Histiocytic Lymphoma; Hodgkin's Lymphoma; Hypertrichosis Lanuginosa

H&L–Heart and Lungs

HLA–Histocompatibility Locus Antigen; Homologous Leukocyte Antibody; Human Leukocyte Antigen; Hypoplastic Left Atrium

HLC–Human Lactation Center

HLD–Herniated Lumbar Disc; Hypersensitivity Lung Disease

HLH–Human Luteinizing Hormone; Hypoplastic Left Heart

HLK–Heart, Liver and Kidneys

HLN–Hyperplastic Liver Nodules

HLP–Hyperlipoproteinemia

HLR–Heart-Lung Resuscitation

HLV–Hypoplastic Left Ventricle

HM–Hand Motion; Hand Movement; Heart Murmur; Heloma Molle; Human Milk; Human Semi-synthetic Insulin; Hydatidiform Mole

Hm–Manifest Hypermetropia; Manifest Hyperopia

HMB–Homatropine Methobromide

HMC–Heroin, Morphine and Cocaine

HMD–Hyaline Membrane Disease
HME–Heat and Moisture Exchanger; Heat, Massage and Exercise
HMG–Human Menopausal Gonadotropin; Hydroxymethylglutaryl
HMI–Healed Myocardial Infarction
HM&LP–Hand Motion and Light Perception
HMM–Hexamethylmelamine
HMO–Heart Minute Output; Health Maintenance Organization
HMP–Hot Moist Packs
HMR–Histiocytic Medullary Reticulosis
HMSAS–Hypertrophic Muscular Subaortic Stenosis
HMT–Human Molar Thyrotropin
HN–Head Nurse; Hereditary Nephritis; Hilar Node; Human Nutrition
HNA–Heparin Neutralizing Activity
HNC–Hypothalamic-Neurohypophyseal Complex
HNP–Herniated Nucleus Pulposus
HNS–Head, Neck and Shaft; Home Nursing Supervisor
HNSHA–Hereditary Nonspherocytic Hemolytic Leukemia
HNV–Has Not Voided
HO–Heterotopic Ossification; High Oxygen; Hyperbaric Oxygen
H/O–Hematology and Oncology; History Of
HOAP–Adriamycin, Cytosine Arabinoside, Vincristine and Prednisone
HOB–Head of Bed
HOC–Human Ovarian Cancer; Hydroxycorticoid
HOCM–Hypertrophic Obstructive Cardiomyopathy
HOD–Hyperbaric Oxygen Drenching
HOG–Halothane, Oxygen and Gas
HOH–Hard of Hearing
HOLD–Hemostatic Occlusive Leverage Device
HOM–Hexamethylmelamine, Oncovin and Methotrexate
HOOD–Hereditary Osteo-Onychodysplasia
HOP–Adriamycin, Vincristine and Prednisone; High Oxygen Pressure
HOPI–History of Present Illness

HOS–Human Osteosarcoma

HOST–Hypo-Osmotic Shock Treatment

HOT–Human Old Tuberculin; Hyperbaric Oxygen Therapy

HP–Handicapped Person; Hemipelvectomy; Hemiplegia; Hexamethylmelamine and Cisplatin; High Potency; High Protein; Highly Purified; Human Pituitary; Hydrophilic Petrolatum; Hyperparathyroidism; Hyperphoria; Hypertension and Proteinuria; Hypopharynx

HPA–Human Papillomavirus; Hypothalamic-Pituitary-Adrenal; Hypothalamic-Pituitary-Adrenocorticoid

HPC–Hippocampal Pyramidal Cell

HPD–Dialysate of Hydropenic Plasma; High Protein Diet; Home Peritoneal Dialysis

HPE–History and Physical Examination

HPF–Heparin-Precipitable Fraction

HPFH–Hereditary Persistance of Fetal Hemoglobin; Human Pituitary Follicle-Stimulating Hormone

HPG–Human Pituitary Gonadotropin

HPI–History of Present Illness

HPLC–High-Performance Liquid Chromatography

HPM–Hemiplegic Migraine

HPN–Home Parenteral Nutrition; Hypertension

HPNS–High-Pressure Nervous Syndrome

HPO–High-Pressure Oxygen; Hydrophilic Ointment; Hypertrophic Pulmonary Osteoarthropathy

HPP–Hereditary Pyropoikilocytosis; Hydroxypyrazolopyrimidine

HPr–Human Prolactin

HPS–High Protein Supplement; Hypertrophic Pyloric Stenosis

HPT–Human Placental Thyrotropin; Hyperparathyroidism

HPV–Hemophilus Pertussis Vaccine; Human Papillomavirus; Hypoxic Pulmonary Vasoconstriction

HPVD–Hypertensive Pulmonary Vascular Disease

HR–Hallux Rigidus; Halstead-Reitan; Harrington Rod; Heart Rate Hemorrhagic Retinopathy; Heterosexual Relations; Hospital Record

H&R–Hysterectomy and Radiation

HRA–Heart Rate Audiometry; Histamine Releasing Activity

HRE–High-Resolution Electrocardiogram

HRI–Harrington Rod Instrumentation

HRIG–Human Rabies Immune Globulin

HRL–Head Rotated Left

HRR–Head Rotated Right; Heart Rate Range

HRRC–Hearing Rehabilitation Research Center

HRS–Hamilton Rating Scale; Hepatorenal Syndrome; Hormone Receptor Site

HS–Half-Strength; Hartman's Solution; Heart Sounds; Heel Spur; Heel Stick; Henoch-Schonlein Syndrome; Hereditary Spherocytosis; Herpes Simplex; Hour of Sleep

H&S–Hysterectomy and Sterilization

HSA–Health Systems Agency; Horse Serum Albumin; Human Serum Albumin; Hypersomnia-Sleep Apnea Syndrome

HSAS–Hypertrophic Subaortic Stenosis

HSBG–Heel Stick Blood Gas

HSC–Hematopoietic Stem Cell

HSE–Herpes Simplex Encephalitis

HSG–Herpes Simplex Genitalis; Hysterosalpingogram

HSGB–Hysterosalpingography

hSGF–Human Skeletal Growth Factor

HSL–Herpes Simplex Labialis

HSM–Hepatosplenomegaly; Holosystolic Murmur

HSN–Hereditary Sensory Neuropathy

HSP–Henoch-Schonlein Purpura; Human Serum Prealbumin

HSRD–Hypertension Secondary to Renal Disease

HSS–Hypertrophic Subaortic Stenosis

HSSE–High Soap Suds Enema

HSTF–Human Serum Thymus Factor

HSV–Herpes Simplex Virus

HSVE–Herpes Simplex Virus Encephalitis

HT–Hammer Toe; Heart Transplant; Home Treatment; Hubbard Tank; Human Thrombin; Hyper-thyroidism; Hypertension; Hypothalamus; Hydrotherapy; Hydroxytryptamine; Hyperopia; Hypermetropia, Total

H&T–Hospitalization and Treatment

HTA–Hypophysiotropic Area

HT–Histologic Technician

HTAT–Human Tetanus Antitoxin

HTB–Hot Tub Bath

HTC–Hepatoma cells; Hypertensive Crisis

HTD–Human Therapeutic Dose

HTF–House Feeding Tube

HTH–Homeostatic Thymus Hormone

HTL–Hearing Threshold Level; Human Thymic Leukemia; Hypermetropia, Left

HTLV–Human T-Cell Leukemia Virus; Human T-Cell Lymphotrophic Virus

HTN–Hypertension

HTO–Heterotopic Ossification; High Tibial Osteotomy; Hospital Transfer Order

HTP–House-Tree-Person Test; Hydroxytryptophan

HTS–Heel-To-Shin Test; Human Thyroid Stimulator

HU–Hemolytic Unit; Hydroxyurea; Hyperemia Unit

HUR–Hydroxyurea

HUS–Hemolytic-Uremic Syndrome; Hyaluronidase Unit for Semen

HV–Hallux Valgus; Has Voided; Hepatic Vein; Herpes Virus; Hyperventilation

H&V–Hemigastrectomy and Vagotomy

HVE–High-Voltage Electrophoresis

HVG–Host Versus Graft

HVR–Hypoxic Ventilatory Response

HVSD–Hydrogen-Detected Ventricular Septal Defect

HW–Heparin Well

HWB–Hot Water Bottle

Hx–History

HXV–Herpes Simplex Virus

Hy–Hypermetropia; Hyperopia; Hypothenar

HYD–Hydroxyurea

HYPP–Hypersegmented Neutrophil

HZ–Herpes Zoster

HZO–Herpes Zoster Ophthalmicus

I

I–Incisal; Impression; Induction; Inspired; Iodine

IA–Image Amplification; Internal Auditory; Intra-Amniotic; Intra-Aortic; Intra-Arterial; Intra-Articular; Intra-Atrial; Intra-Auricular

I&A–Irrigation and Aspiration

IAA–International Antituberculosis Association; Interrupted Aortic Arch

IAB–Intra-Abdominal; Intra-Aortic Balloon

IABC–Intra-Aortic Balloon Catheter; Intra-Aortic Balloon Counterpulsation

IABP–Intra-Aortic Balloon Pump

IAC–Internal Auditory Canal; Intra-Arterial Chemotherapy; Isolated Adrenal Cell

IACB–Intraaortic Counterpulsation Balloon

IAC-CPR–Interposed Abdominal Compressions-Cardiopulmonary Resuscitation

IAD–Internal Absorbed Dose

IADH–Inappropriate Antidiuretic Hormone

IA DSA–Intra-Arterial Digital Subtraction Arteriography

IAE–Intra-Atrial Electrocardiogram

IAFI–Infantile Amaurotic Familial Idiocy

IAHD–Idiopathic Acquired Hemolytic Disease

IAI–Intra-Abdominal Infection

IAM–Internal Acoustic Meatus; Internal Auditory Meatus

I&O–Intake and Output

IAO–Immediately After Onset; Intermittent Aortic Occlusion

IAP–Intermittent Acute Porphyria

IAS–Interatrial Septum; Intra-Amniotic Saline

IASD–Interatrial Septal Defect

IAT–Iowa Achievement Test

IAV–Intra-Arterial Vasopressin

IB–Infectious Bronchitis; Isolation Bed

IBB–Intestinal Brush Border

IBC–Iron-Binding Capacity

IBD–Inflammatory Bowel Disease; Ischemic Bowel Disease

IBF–Immunoglobin-Binding Factor

IBI–Intermittent Bladder Irrigation

IBK–Infectious Bovine Keratoconjunctivitis

IBPMS–Indirect Blood Pressure Measuring System

IBR–Infectious Bovine Rhinotracheitis

IBS–Irritable Bowel Syndrome

IBV–Infectious Bronchitis Vaccine

IC–Icteric; Ileocecal; Iliococcygeal; Iliocostal; Indirect Calorimetry; Individual Counseling; Inferior Colliculus; Inspiratory Center; Intercostal; Intermittent Catheterization; Intermittent Claudication; Internal Capsule; Internal Carotid; Internal Cerebral; Internal Cholecystectomy; Internal Conjugate; Intracarotid; Intracardiac; Intracerebral; Intracisternal; Intracranial; Intrapleural Catheter; Irritable Colon; Islet Cells; Isovolumic Contraction

ICA–Internal Carotid Artery; Intracranial Aneurysm

ICAO–Internal Carotid Artery Occlusion

ICBT–Intercostobronchial Trunk

ICC–Indian Childhood Cirrhosis; Intensive Coronary Care; Internal Conversion Coefficient

ICCE–Intracapsular Cataract Extraction

ICCM–Idiopathic Congestive Cardiomyopathy

ICCU–Intensive Coronary Care Unit

ICD–Immune Complex Disease; Instantaneous Cardiac Death; Intrauterine Contraceptive Device

ICF–Indirect Centrifugal Flotation; Intracellular Fluid; Intravascular Coagulation and Fibrinolysis

ICH–Infectious Canine Hepatitis; Intracranial Hemorrhage

ICJ–Ileocecal Junction

ICLE–Intracapsular Lens Extraction

ICM–Infracostal Margin; Intercostal Margin

ICN–Intensive Care Nursery

ICP–Infection-Control Practitioner; Intracranial Pressure

ICPP–Intubated Continuous Positive Pressure; Isochromic Color Perception Plates

ICR–Distance Between Iliac Crests; Intensive Care Room; Intracranial Reinforcement

ICS–Intracellular-Like Solution; Intracranial Stimulation

ICSH–Interstitial Cell-Stimulating Hormone

ICT–Icterus; Inflammation of Connective Tissue; Insulin Coma Therapy; Intermittent Cervical Traction; Isovolumic Contraction Time

ICU–Intensive Care Unit

ICV–Intracrebroventricular

ICVH–Ischemic Cerebrovascular Headache

ICW–Intracellular Water

ID–Immunodeficiency; Inclusion Disease; Infant Deaths; Infectious Disease; Infective Dose; Intradermal; Intraduodenal

I&D–Incision and Drainage; Irrigation and Debridement; Irrigation and Drainage

IDA–Iron Deficiency Anemia

IDCF–Immunodiffusion Complement Fixation

IDDM–Insulin-Dependent Diabetes Mellitus

IDDS–Implantable Drug Delivery System

ID/ED–Internal Diameter to External Diameter

IDFC–Immature Dead Female Child

IDI–Induction-Delivery Interval

IDIC–Internal Dose Information Center

IDK–Internal Derangement of Knee

IDM–Idiopathic Disease of the Myocardium; Infant of Diabetic Mother

IDMC–Immature Dead Male Child

IDP–Initial Dose Period; Instantaneous Diastolic Pressure

IDPH–Idiopathic Pulmonary Hemosiderosis

IDR–Intradermal Reaction

IDS–Immunity Deficiency State; Incremented Dynamic Scanning

IDSA–Intraoperative Digital Subtraction Angiography

IDU–Idoxuridine; Iododeoxyuridine

IDV–Intermittent Demand Ventilation

IDVC–Indwelling Venous Catheter

IE–Intake Energy

IEA–Intravascular Erythrocyte Aggregation

IEC–Injection Electrode Catheter; Inpatient Exercise Center; Intraepithelial Carcinoma

IEE–Inner Enamel Epithelium

IEMG–Integrated Electromyogram

IF–Immunofluorescence; Internal Fixation; Interstitial Fluid; Involved Field

IFM–Intrafusal Muscle

IFR–Inspiratory Flow Rate

IFV–Intracellular Fluid Volume

IG–Immunoglobulin; Intragastric

IGDM–Infant of Gestational Diabetic Mother

IGF–Insulin-Like Growth Factor

IGH–Idiopathic Growth Hormone; Immunoreactive Growth Hormone

IGIV–Immune Globulin Intravenous

IGR–Intrauterine Growth Retardation

IGS–Inappropriate Gonadotropin Secretion

IGT–Impaired Glucose Tolerance

IGV–Intrathoracic Gas Volume

IH–Immediate Hypersensitivity; Infectious Hepatitis; Inguinal Hernia

IHA–Infusion Hepatic Arteriography

IHAS–Idiopathic Hypertrophic Aortic Stenosis

IHB–Incomplete Heart Block

IHBTD–Incompatible Hemolytic Blood Transfusion Disease

IHC–Idiopathic Hypercalciuria; Idiopathic Hemochromatosis; Immobilization Hypercalcemia

IHD–Intrahepatic Duct; Ischemic Heart Disease

IHH–Idiopathic Hypogonadotropic Hypogonadism

IHO–Idiopathic Hypertrophic Osteoarthropathy

IHOP–Adriamycin, Isophosphamide, Vincristine and Prednisone

IHP–Idiopathic Hypoparathyroidism; Inverted Hand Position

IHPH–Intrahepatic Portal Hypertension

IHR–Intrahepatic Resistance; Intrinsic Heart Rate

Ihs–Iris Hamartoma

IHSS–Idiopathic Hypertrophic Subaortic Stenosis

IHT–Insulin Hypoglycemia test; Intravenous Histamine Test

IHW–Inner Heel Wedge

IICP–Increased Intracranial Pressure

IICU–Infant Intensive Care Unit

ILA–Insulin-Like Activity

ILBW–Infant Low Birth Weight

ILC–Incipient Lethal Concentration

ILD–Interstitial Lung Disease; Ischemic Leg Disease; Ischemic Limb Disease

ILFC–Immature Living Female Child

ILL–Intermediate Lymphocytic Lymphoma

ILM–Insulin-Like Material; Internal Limiting Membrane

ILMC–Immature Living Male Child

ILMI–Inferolateral Myocardial Infarction

ILMN–Incomplete Lower Motor Neuron

IM–Infectious Mononucleosis; Intermetatarsal; Intermuscular; Internal Medicine; Internal Monitor; Intramedullary; Intramuscular; Invasive Mole

IMA–Inferior Mesenteric Artery; Internal Mammary Artery

IMAA–Iodinated Macroaggregated Albumin

IMAG–Internal Mammary Artery Graft

IMB–Intermenstrual Bleeding

IMBC–Indirect Maximum Breathing Capacity

IMD–Immunologically Mediated Diseases

IMF–Intermaxillary Fixation

IMG–Inferior Mesenteric Ganglion

IMH–Idiopathic Myocardial Hypertrophy; Indirect Microhemagglutination Test

IMI–Inferior Myocardial Infarction; Intramuscular Injection

IMIG–Intramuscular Immunoglobulin

IMPA–Incisal Mandibular Plane Angle

IMR–Infant Mortality Rate

IMRAD–Introduction, Methods, Results and Discussion

IMSS–In-Flight Medical Support System

IMT–Induced Muscular Tension

IMTLYM–Immature Lymphocytes

IMV–Inferior Mesenteric Vein; Intermittent Mandatory Ventilation; Isophosphamide, Vincristine and Methotrexate

IN–Icterus Neonatorum; Interneuron; Intranasal

INAD–Infantile Neuroaxonal Dystrophy

INC–Incontinent; Inside-the-Needle Catheter

INCS–Incomplete Resolution, Scan to Follow

IND–Investigational New Drug

INDM–Infant of Nondiabetic Mother

INE–Infantile Necrotizing Encephalomyelopathy

INFM–Infectious Mononucleosis

INH–Isonicotine Hydrazine

INI–Intranuclear Inclusion

INO–Intranuclear Ophthalmoplegia

INPH–Iproniazid Phosphate

INPRONS–Information Processing in the Central Nervous System

INPV–Intermittent Negative-Pressure Assisted Ventilation

INREM–Internal Radiation Dose

INS–Idiopathic Nephrotic Syndrome

INSU–Intensive Neurosurgery Unit

INTH–Intrathecal

IO–Incisal Opening; Inferior Oblique; Initial Opening; Internal Os; Intestinal Obstruction; Intraocular

IOCG–Intraoperative Cholecystogram

IOD–Interorbital Distance

IODA–Iron Overload Diseases Association

IODM–Infant of Diabetic Mother

IOF–Intraocular Fluid

IOH–Idiopathic Orthostatic Hypotension

IOL–Intraocular Lens

ION–Ischemic Optic Neuropathy

IORT–Intraoperative Radiation Therapy

IOS–Intraoperative Sonography

IOT–Intraocular Tension; Intraocular Transfer; Ipsilateral Optic Tectum

IP–Icterus Praecox; Iliopsoas; Incisoproximal; Incisopulpal; Incubation Period; Induction Period; Infection Prevention; Infundibulopelvic; Initial Pressure; Intraperitoneal; Isoelectric Point

IPA–Invasive Pulmonary Aspergillosis

IPC–Interpenduncular Cistern

IPCD–Infantile Polycystic Disease

IPCS–Intrauterine Progesterone Contraceptive System

IPD–Inflammatory Pelvic Disease; Intermittent Peritoneal Dialysis; Inventory of Psychosocial Development

IPE–Initial Psychiatric Evaluation

IPEH–Intravascualr Papillary Endothelial Hyperplasia

IPF–Idiopathic Pulmonary Fibrosis

IPFD–Intrapartum Fetal Distress

IPG–Impedance Plethysmography; Inspiratory Gas Phase

IPGE–Immunoreactive Prostaglandin E

IPH–Idiopathic Pulmonary Hemosiderosis; Interphalangeal

IPK–Interphalangeal Keratosis; Intractable Plantar Keratosis

IPMI–Inferoposterior Myocardial Infarction

IPN–Infantile Periarteritis Nodosa; Interpeduncular Nucleus

IPP–Inferior Point of the Pubic; Inflatable Penile Prosthesis; Intermittent Positive Pressure; Intrapleural Pressure

IPPA–Inspection, Palpation, Percussion and Auscultation

IPPB–Intermittent Positive Pressure Breathing

IPPO–Intermittent Positive Pressure Inflation with Oxygen

IPPR–Intermittent Positive Pressure Respiration

IPPV–Intermittent Positive Pressure Ventilation

IPQ–Intimacy Potential Quotient

IPRT–Interpersonal Reaction Test

IPS–Infundibular Pulmonic Stenosis; Intermittent Photic Stimulation; Intraperitoneal Shock

IPSID–Immunoproliferative Small Intestinal Disease

IPSP–Inhibitory Postsynaptic Potential

IPT–Intermittent Pelvic Traction

IPTH–Immunoreactive Parathyroid Hormone

IPV–Inactivated Poliomyelitis Vaccine; Infectious Pustular Vaginitis; Infectious Pustular Vulvovaginitis

IR–Immune Response; Inferior Rectus; Intelligence Ratio; Internal Rotation

IRBBB–Incomplete Right Bundle-Branch Block

IRC–Infrared Coagulator; Inspiratory Reserve Capacity

IRDS–Idiopathic Respiratory Distress Syndrome; Infant Respiratory Distress Syndrome

IRE–Internal Rotation in Flexion

IRG–Immunoreactive Glucagon

IRGH–Immunoreactive Growth Hormone

IRHCS–Immunoradioassayable Human Chorionic Somatomammotropin

IRI–Immunoreactive Insulin

IRMA–Immunoradiometric Assay; Intraretinal Microangiopathy; Intraretinal Microvascular Abnormalities

IROS–Ipsilateral Routing of Signal

IRR–Intrarenal Reflux

IRS–Instument Retrieval System

IRSA–Idiopathic Refractory Sideroblastic Anemia

IRT–Isometric Relaxation Time; Instrument Retrieval Containers

IRV–Inspiratory Reserve Volume

IS–Incentive Spirometry; Induced Sputum; Intercostal Space; Intraspinal

ISA–Iodinated Serum Albumin

ISADH–Inappropriate Secretion of Antidiuretic Hormone

ISB–Incentive Spirometry Breathing

ISC–Irreversibly Sickled Cell

ISD–Inhibited Sexual Desire; Isosorbide Dinitrate

ISE–Inhibited Sexual Excitement

ISF–Interstitial Fluid

ISG–Immune Serum Globulin

ISH–Icteric Serum Hepatitis; Inner Self Helper; Isolated Systolic Hypertension

ISI–Infarct Size Index; Injury Severity Index

ISM–Intersegmental Muscles

ISMA–Infantile Spinal Muscular Atrophy

ISP–Interspinal

ISR–Integrated Secretory Response

IST–Insulin Shock Therapy

ISY–Intrasynovial

IT–Iliotibial; Inferior Turbinate; Inhalation Test; Inspiratory Time; Intertrochanteric; Intradermal Test; Intrathecal; Intratracheal; Intratracheal Tube; Ischial Tuberosity

ITCP–Idiopathic Thrombocytopenic Purpura

ITE–Insufficient Therapeutic Effect; In The Ear

ITP–Idiopathic Thrombocytopenic Purpura

ITR–Intraocular Tension Recorder; Intratracheal

ITT–Iliotibial Tract; Insulin Tolerance Test; Internal Tibial Torsion

ITVAD–Indwelling Transcutaneous Vascular Access Device

IUC–Idiopathic Ulcerative Colitis

IUCD–Intrauterine Contraceptive Device; Intrauterine Death

IUFD–Intrauterine Fetal Death

IUFGR–Intrauterine Fetal Growth Retardation

IUGR–Intrauterine Growth Rate

IUM–Intrauterine Fetally Malnourished

IUP–Intrauterine Pregnancy; Intrauterine Pressure

IUT–Intrauterine Transfusion

IV–Interventricular; Intervertebral; Intravascular; Intravenously; Intraventricular; Intravertebral

IVAC–Intravenous Accurate Control

IVBAT–Intravascular Bronchoalveolar Tumor

IVC–Inferior Vena Cava; Inferior Venacavogram; Inspiratory Vital Capacity; Intravenous Cholangiogram; Intraventricular Catheter; Isovolumic Contraction

IVCC–Intravascular Consumption Coagulopathy

IVCD–Interventricular Conduction Delay

IVCh–Intravenous Cholangiogram

IVCP–Inferior Vena Cava Pressure

IVCU–Isotope-Voiding Cystourethrogram

IVCV–Inferior Venacavography

IVD–Intervertebral Disk

IVF–Intravascular Fluid; In Vitro Fertilization

IVG–Isotopic Ventriculogram

IVH–Intravenous Hyperalimentation; Intraventricular Hemorrhage

IVJC–Intervertebral Joint Complex

IVLBW–Infant of Very Low Birth Weight

IVM–Intravascular Mass

IVN–Intravenous Nutrition

IVP–Intravenous Pitocin; Intravenous Pyelogram

IVPF–Isovolume Pressure Flow

IVR–Idioventricular Rhythm; Internal Visual Reference

IVSD–Interventricular Septal Defect

IVT–Intravenous Transfusion; Intraventricular

IVU–Intravenous Urogram

IVV–Intravenous Vasopressin

IWMI–Inferior Wall Myocardial Infarction

IZS–Insulin Zinc Suspension

J

J–Juvenile; Joint

JA–Juvenile Atrophy; Juxta-Articular

JAI–Juvenile Amaurotic Idiocy
JAMG–Juvenile Autoimmune Myasthenia Gravis
JBC–Jesness Behavior Checklist
JBE–Japanese B Encephalitis
JC–Jakob-Creutzfeldt
JCA–Juvenile Chronic Arthritis
JCAH–Joint Commission on Accreditation of Hospitals
JCC–Joint Commission on Contraception
JCF–Juvenile Calcaneal Fracture
JCM–Juvenile Chronic Myelocytic
JCML–Juvenile Chronic Myelocytic Leukemia
JD–Jejunal Diverticulitis; Jugulodigastric Node; Juvenile Diabetes
JDM–Juvenile-Onset Diabetes mellitus
JDMS–Juvenile Dermatomyositis
JE–Japanese Encephalitis; Junctional Escape
JEE–Japanese Equine Encephalitis
JEJ–Jejunum
JF–Joint Fluid; Jugular Foramen; Junctional Fold
JFS–Jugular Foramen Syndrome
JGA–Juxtaglomerular Apparatus
JGCT–Juxtaglomerular Cell Tumor
JGI–Jejunogastric Intussusception; Juxtaglomerular Granulation Index
JGP–Juvenile General Paralysis
JHA–Juvenile Hormone Analogue
JHR–Jarisch-Herxheimer Reaction
JI–Jejunoileal; Jejunoileostomy
JLP–Juvenile Laryngeal Papilloma
JM–Jugomaxillary
JODM–Juvenile-Onset Diabetes Mellitus
JOMAC–Judge, Orientation, Memory, Abstraction, and Calculation
JP–Jackson Pratt (drain); Jobst Pump; Juvenile Periodontitis
JPB–Junctional Premature Beat

JPC–Junctional Premature Contraction

JPD–Juvenile Plantar Dermatosis

JPI–Jacson Personality Inventory

JPS–Joint Position Sense

JR–Jolly's Reaction; Junctional Rhythm; Juveline Rheumatoid Arthritis

JRA–Juvenile Rheumatoid Arthritis

JS–Jejunal Segment; Junctional Slowing; Junkman-Schoeller

JSI–Jansky Screening Index

JVD–Jugular Venous Distention

JVIS–Jackson Vocational Interest Survey

JVP–Jugular Vein Pulse

JVPT–Jugular Venous Pulse Tracing

JXG–Juvenile Xanthogranuloma

K

K–Absolute Zero; Coefficient of Scleral Rigidity; Kelvin; Kidney; Kirschner; Knee;

KA–Kathode; Keratoacanthoma; Ketoacidosis

KAB–Knowledge, Attitude, Behavior

KABC–Kaufman Assessment Battery for Children

KAFO–Knee-Ankle-Foot Orthosis

KAFO's–Knee-Ankle-Foot Orthoses

KAP–Knowledge, Attitudes, and Practice

KAS–Katz Adjustment Scale

KAST–Kindergarten Auditory Screening Test

KB–Kashin-Beck; Knee Brace

Kb Splint–Knuckle-Bender Splint

KC–Keratoconus; Keratoma Climacterium; Knees to Chest; Knuckle Cracking; Kupffer Cells

KCC–Kathodal Closing Contraction

KCCT–Kaolin-Cephalin Clotting Time
KCG–Kinetocardiogram
DCS–Keratoconjunctivitis Sicca
KD–Kawaasaki's Disease; Keto-Diastix; Knee Disarticulation
KDSM–Keratizing Desquamative Squamous Metaplasia
KERV–Kentucky Equine Respiratory Virus
KF–Kidney Function; Klippel-Feil
KFAO–Knee-Foot-Ankle Orthosis
KFDT–Kinetic Family Drawing Test
KFS–Klippel-Feil Syndrome
KGC–Keflin, Gentamycin, and Carbenicillin
KGHT–Kidney Glodblatt Hypertension
KGS–Ketogenci Steroid
KID–Keratitis, Ichthyosis, and Deafness
KIDS–Kent Infant Development Scale
KIMSV–Kirsten Murine Sarcoma Virus
KISS–Key Integrative Social System; Saturated Solution of Potassium
    Iodide
KIU–Kallikrein Inactivation Unit
kj–Knee Jerk
KK–Knee Kick
KKK–Kolmer, Kline, Kahn
KL–Kidney Lobe; Kleine-Levine Syndrome
KLS–Kidney(s), Liver, and Spleen
KLST–Kindergarten Language Screening Test
KM–Kraepelin-Morel Disease
KMDAT–Key Math Diagnostic Arithmetic Test
KMV–Killed Measles Virus Vaccine
KNL–Darrow's Solution
KNO–Keep Needle Open
KO–Keep On; Keep Open; Knee Orthhosis; Knocked Out
KOT–Knowledge of Occupations Test

KP–Keratitic Precipitates; Keratitis Punctata; Keratoprecipitate; Kidney Protein; Killed Parenteral

KPE–Kelman Phakoemulsification

KP's–Keratitic Precipitates; Keratoprecipitates

KPPT–Kaolin Partial Thromboplastin Time

KPV–Killed Parenteral Vaccine

KRA–Klinefelter-Reifenstein-Albright

KS–Kaposi's Ssarcoma; Kartagener's Syndrome; Klinefelter's Syndrome; Kugel-Stoloff Syndrome;

Kugel-Stoloff Syndrome; Kveim-Siltzbach Test

KSA–Knowledge, Skills, and Abilities

KSC–Kathodal (Obsolete for Cathodal Closing) Contraction

KSP–Kidney-Specific Protein

KT–Kidney Transplant; Klippel Trenaunay Syndrome; Kuder Test

KTS–Kiersley Temperament Sorter

KTSA–Kahn Test of Symbol Arrangement

KTU–Kidney Transplant Unit

KUB–Kidney and Upper Bladder; Kindey(s), Ureter(s), and Bladder

KUF–Kidney Ultrafiltration Rate

KV–Kanamycin-Vancomycin; Killed Virus

KVE–Kaposi's Varicelliform Eruption

KVO–Keep Vein Open

KW–Keith–Wagner Test; Kimmelstiel-Wilson Syndrom; Kugelberg-Welander Disease

KWB–Keith, Wagener, Barker

KWE–Keith-Welti-Ernst Method

L

L–Left Eye; Lente Insulin; Lethal; Lidocaine; Ligament; Light Sense; Lingual; Liver; Lumbar; Lumen; Lung; Lymphogranuloma

LA–Left Angle; Left Angulation; Left Arm; Left Atrial; Left Atrium; Left Auricle; Left Antigen; Lichen Amyloidosis; Linguoaxial; Linoleic Acid; Lobuloalveolar; Local Anesthesia; Long-Arm Cast; Low Anxiety; Ludwig's Angina

L & A–Light and Accommodation; Living and Active

La–Labial

LAA–Left Atrial Abnormalities; Left Atrial Appendage; Leukemia-Associated Antigen

LABVT–Left Atrial Ball-Valve Thrombus

LAC–Laceration; La Crosse Subtype Encephalitis; Lactose; Left Atrial Contraction; Lingoaxiocervical; Long-Arm Cast; Low Amplitude Contraction

LAD–Language Acquistion Device; Left Anterior Descending; Left Axis Deviation

LADA–Laboratory Animal Dander Allergy; Left Acromiodorsoanterior; Left Anterior Descending Artery

LADCA–Left Anterior Descending Coronary Artery

LADD–Left Anterior Descending Diagonal

LADME–Liberation, Absorption, Distribution, Metabolism, Excertion

LADP–Left Acromiodorsoposterior

LADu–Lobuloalveolar-Ductal

LAE–Left Atrial Enlargement; Long Above–Elbow Cast

LAF–Laminar Airflow; Latin American Female; Leukocyte-Activating Factor; Lymphocyte-Activating Factor

LAFB–Left Anterior Ffascicular Block

LAG–Labiogingival; Linguoaxiogingival; Lymphangiogram

LAH–Left Anterior Hemiblock; Left Atrial Hypertrophy

Lal–Labioincisal

LAL–Left Axillary Line

LAM–L-Asparaginase and Methotrexate; Late Ambulatory Monitoring; Latin American Male; Left Atrial Myxoma; Lymphangioleiomyomatosis

Lam–Laminectomy; Lamingram

LAN–Long-Acting Neuroleptic; Lymmphadenopathy

LANC–Long-Arm Navicular Cast

LANV–Left Atrial Neovascularization

LAO–Left Anterior Oblique; Left Anterior Occiptal Position; Left Atrial Overloading;

LAP–Left Arterial Presure; Left Atrial Pressure; Lyophilized Anterior Pituitary

LAPMS–Long Arm Posterior Molded Splint

LAPOCA–L-Asparaginase, Prednisone, Vincristine, Cytosine Arabinoside and Adriamycin

LAPSE–Long-Term Ambulatory Physiological Surveillance

LAPW–Left Posterior Wall

LAR–Laryngology; Late Asthmatic Response; Left Arm Recumbent;

LARS–Language-Structured Auditory Retention Span Test

LAS–Laxative Abuse Syndrome; Left Anterior-Superior; Left Arm Sitting; Local Adaptation Syndrome; Long-Arm Splint; Lower Abdominal Surgery; Lymphadenopathy Syndrome

LASFB–Left Anterior-Superior Fascicular Block

LASH–Left Anterosuperior Hemiblock;

LASS–Linguistic Analysis of Speech Samples

LAT–Left Anterior Thigh

LATCH–Literature Attached to Charts

LATS–Long-Acting Thyroid Stimulating Hormone

LAV–Lymphadenopathy-Associated Virus

LB–Large Bowel; Left Breast; Left Buttock; Leiomyoblastoma; Live Births; Loose Body; Low Back;

L & B–Left and Below

LBB–Left Breast Biopsy

LBBB–Left Bundle-Branch Block

LBCD–Left Border of Cardiac Dullness

LBF–Lactobacillus Bulgaricus Factor; Liver Blood Flow;

LBH–Length, Breadth, and Height
LBI–Low Serum-Bound Iron
LBL–Lymphoblastic Lymphoma
LBM–Lean Body Mass
LBO–Large Bowel Obstruction
LBP–Low Back Pain; Low Blood Pressure
LBS–Low Back Strain
LBV–Left Brachial Vein
LBW–Low Birth Weight
LBWI–Low Birth Weight Infant
LBWR–Lung-Body Weight Ratio
LC–Laennec's Cirrhosis; Lethal Concentration; Linguocervical; Living Children
LCA–Leber's Congenital Amaurosis; Left Carotid Artery; Left Coronary Artery
LCAR–Late Cutaneous Anaphylactic Reaction
LCCA–Left Circumflex Coronary Artery; Left Common Carotid Artery; Leukocytoclastic Angitis;
LCCS–Low Cervical Cesarean Section
LCD–Localized Collagen Dystrophy
LCF–Left Common Femoral Artery
LCL–Lateral Colateral Ligament; Levinthal-Coles-Lillie; Lymphocytic Leukemia; Lymphocytic Lymphosarcoma
LCLC–Large Cell Lung Carcinoma
LCM–Left Costal Margin; Lymphatic Choriomeningitis
LCP–Legge-Calve-Perthes Disease
LCR–Late Cutaneous Reaction; Leurocristine
LCS–Lichen Chronicus Simplex; Low Constant Suction; Low Continuous Suction
LCT–Luscher Color Test
L.C.T.–Low Cervicla Transverse
LCV–Low Cervical Vertical

LCX–Left Circumflex Coronary Artery

LD–Labor and Delivery; Labyrinthine Defect; Lactate Dehydrogenase; Left Deltoid; Legionnarie's Disease; Lethal Dose; Levodopa; Light Difference; Linguodistal; Liver Disease; Living Donor; Loading Dose; Low Density; Low Dosage

LDA–Left Dorsoanterior Position

LDD–Light-Dark Discrimination

LDHI–Lactic Dehydrogenase Isoenzymes

LDL–Loudness Discomfort Level; Low-Density Lipoprotein

L-DOPA–Levodopa

LDS–Licentiate in Dental Surgery; Ligating and Dividing Stapler

LDUB–Long Double Upright Brace

LDV–Laser Doppler Velocimetry

LE–Left Eye; Lower Extremity; Lupus Erythematosus

LEHPZ–Lower Esoophageal High Pressure Zone

LEL–Lowest Effect Level

LEM–Lateral Eye Movements

LEOD–Lens Extraction, Oculus Dexter

LEOS–Lens Extraction, Oculus Sinister

LEP–Lupus Erythematosus Preparation

LES–Lateral Epithelial Space; Local Excitatory State; Lower Esophageal Sphincter; Systemic Lupus Erythematosus

LESS–Lateral Electrical Spine Stimulation

LESP–Lower Esophageal Sphincter Pressure

LEVT–Left Extremity Venous Tracing; Lower Extremity Venous Tracing

LF–Laryngofissure; Left Foot; Low Forceps; Low Frequency;

LFA–Left Femoral Artery; Left Frontoanterior; Low Friction Arthroplasty

LFC–Living Female Child

LFD–Least Fatal Dose; Low-Fat Diet; Low Forceps Delivery

LFH–Left Femoral Hernia

LFOV–Large Field of View
LFP–Left Frontoposterior
LFT–Left Frontotransverse; Liver Function Tests
LG–Laryngectomy; Left Gluteus; Linguogingival
LGA–Large for Gestational Age
LGB–Landry-Guillain-Barre
LGd–Dorsolateral Geniculate
LGL–Labioglossolaryngeal; Lown-Ganong-Levine
LGN–Lobular Glomerulonephritis
LGP–Labioglossopharyngeal
LGS–Large Green Soft Stool
LGT–Langat Encephalitis; Late Generalized Tuberculosis
LGV–Lymphogranuloma Venerum
LG–Left Hand; Left Hyperphoria; Lues Hereditaria; Luteinizing Hormone
LGC–Left Hypochondrium
LHF–Left Heart Failure
LHL–Left Hemisphere Lesion; Left Hepatic Lobe
Lhp–Left Hemiparesis
LHRF–Luteinizing Hormone-Releasing Factor
LGS–Left Hand Side; Left Heart Strain
Lht–Left Hypertropia;
LI–Left Iliac; Linguoincisal; Low Impulsivenes
LIA–Leukemia–Associated Inhibitory Activity; Lock-In Amplifier
LIAFI–Late Infantile Amaurotic Idiocy
LIB–Left In Bottle
LIBC–Latent Iron-Binding Capacity
LIC–Left Iliac Crest; Left Internal Carotid Artery; Limiting Isorrheic Concentration
LICA–Left Internal Carotid Artery
LICM–Left Intercostal Margin
LICS–Lieft Intercostal Space

LIF–Left Iliac Fossa

Lih–Left Inguinal Hernia

LIHA–Low Impulsiveness,High Anxiety

LILA–Low Impulsivenes,Low Anxiety

LIMA–Left Internal Mammary Artery

LIO–Left Inferior Oblique

L.I.P.–Lymphocytic Interstitial Pneumonia

LIPT–Leiter International Performance Test

LIQ–Lower Inner Quadrant

LIR–Left Iliac Region

LIRBM–Liver, Iron, Red Bone Marrow

LIS–Left Intercostal Space; Lobular In Situ; Low Intermittent Suction;

LIV–Left Innominate Vein; Liver Battery Test

LJL–Lateral Joint Line

LK–Left Kidney

LKS–Liver, Kidneys, and Spleen

LKV–Lengyel-Kerman-Vargar

LL–Left Lateral; Left Leg; Left Lung; Lower Leg; Lower Lid; Lower
   Lip; Lower Lobe; Lumbar Length; Lymphoblastic Lymphoma

LLB–Long Leg Brace

LLBCD–Left Lower Border of Cardiac Dullnes

LLC–Long-Leg Cast; Lymphocytic Leudemia, Chronic

LLD–Leg Length Discrepancy

LLE–Left Lower Extremity

LLF–Laki-Lorand Factor; Left Lateral Femoral

LL-GXT–Low-Level Graded Exercise Test

LLL–Left Lower Lid; Left Lower Limb; Left Lower Lobe: Left Lower
   Lung

LLQ–Left Lower Quadrant

LLR–Left Lateral Rectus; Left Lumbar Region

LLS–Lazy Leukocyte Syndrome; Long Leg Spling

LLSB–Left Lower Sternal Border

LLT–Left Lateral; Left Lateral Thigh

LLWC–Long-Leg Walking Cast

LM–Labiomental; Laryngeal Muscle; Lateral Malleolus; Licentiate in Midwifery; Light Minimum; Linguomesial; Lipid Mobilizing Hormone; Longitudinal Muscle; Lower Motor Neuron

LMA–Left Mentoanterior; Liver Membrane Autoantibody

LMB–Laurence-Moon-Biedl Syndrome; Leiomyoblastoma

LMC–Living Male Child

LMCA–Left Main Coronary Artery; Left Middle Cerebral Artery

LMD–Low Molecular Weight Dextran

LME–Left Mediolateral Episiotomy

LMEE–Left Middle Ear Exploration

LMF–Chlorambucil, Methotrexate and 5-Fluo-Rouracil

LML–Left Mediolateral Episiotomy; Left Middle Lobe of Ling

LMM–Lentgo Maligna Melanoma

LMN–Lower Motor Neuron

LMP–Last Menstrual Period; Left Mentoposterior Position; Lumbar Puncture

LMR–Left Medial Rectus

LMS–Leiomyosarcoma

LMT–Left Mentotransverse

LN–Labionasal; Lipoid Nephrosis; Lupus Nephritis; Lymph Node

LNB–Lymph Node Biopsy

LND–Lymph Node Dissection

LNMP–Last Normal Menstrual Period

LNNB–Luria-Nebraska Neuropsychological Battery

LNR–Lymph Node Region

LO–Lateral Oblique; Lenticular Opacity; Linguo-Occlusal; Love Object

LOA–Left Anterior Oblique; Left Occipitoanterior

LOC–Laxative of Choice; Level of Care; Level of Consciousness; Loss of Consciousness

LOF–Low Outlet Forceps

LOL–Left Occipitolateral Position

LOM–Left Otitis Media; Liimitation of Motion; Loss of Motion

LOMSA–Left Otitis Media Suppurative Acute

LOMSCh–Left Otitis Media Suppurative Chronic

LOP–Left Occipitoposterior

LOQ–Lower Outer Quadrant

LOS–Length of Stay; Low Output Syndrome

LOT–Left Occipitotransverse

LOWBI–Low-Birth-Weight Infant

LP–Laryngeal-Pharyngeal; Latency Period; Latent Period; Light Perception; Linguoopulpal; Low Protein; Lumbar-Peritoneal; Lumbar Punctar

LPA–Left Pulmonary Artery

LPAM–L-Phenylalanine

L-PAM–L-Phenylalanine Mustard; L-Phenylalanine, Procarbazine, Adriamycin, and Methotrexate

LPC–Laser Photocoagulation

LPD–Luteal Phase Defect

LPE–Lipoprotein Electrophoresis

LPF–Leukocytosis-Promoting Factor; Localized Plaque Formation; Lympocytosis-Promoting Factor

LPH–Left Posterior Hemiblock; Lipotropic Pituitary Hormone

LPM–Liters Per Minute

LPO–Hypothalamic-Pituitary-Ovarian; Left Posterior Oblique; Left Posterior Ocipital; Light Perception Only; Lobus Parolfactorius

LPS–Lanterman-Petris Short Act; Last Papanicolaou Smear

LPV–Left Pulmonary Vein; Lymphopathia Venereum

LQ–Lordosis Quotient

LR–Labor Room; Lactated Ringer's; Latency Relaxation; Lateral Rectus; Light Reaction

LRA–Left Renal Artery

LRC–Lower Rib Cage

LRD–Living Related Donor; Living Renal Donor

L.R.E.–Least Restrictive Environment

LRF–Luteinizing Hormone-Releasing Factor

LRM–Left Radical Mastectomy

LRND–Left Radical Neck Dissection

LRQ–Lower Right Quadrant

LRR–Labyrinthine Righting Reflex

LRS–Lactated Ringer's Solution; Lights Retention Scale

LRT–Lower Respiratory Tract

LRTI–Lower Respiratory Tract Illness

LRV–Left Renal Vein

LS–Lateral Suspensor Ligament; Left Sacrum; Leiomyosarcoma; Liminal Sensation; Liminal Sensitivity; Liver and Spleen; Lumbosacral; Lymphosarcoma

L/S–Lecithin/Sphingomyelin Ratio

LSA–Language Sampling Analysis; Left Sacroanterior; Lichen Sclerosis Et Atrophicus; Lymphosarcoma

L.S.A.–Left Sacroanterior Position;

LSA/RCS–Lymphosarcoma-Reticulum Cell Sarcoma;

LSB–Left Sternal Border

LS BPS–Laparoscopic Bilateral Partial Salpingectomies

LSC–Late Systolic Click; Left-Side Colon; Lid(s), Sclera(e), and Conjuctiva(e)

LSCA–Left Subclavian Artery

LScA–Left Scapuloanterior Position

LSCS–Lower Segment Cesarean Section

LSCV–Left Subclavian Vein

LSD–Lysergic Acid Diethylamide; Low-Salt Diet

LSE–Left Sternal Edge; Local Side Effects

LSF–Low Saturated Fat; Lymphocyte-Stimulating Factor

LSH–Lutein Stimulating Hormone; Lymphocyte-Stimulating Hormone

LSK–Liver, Spleen, and Kidney(s)

LSKM–Liver-Spleen-Kidney-Megaly

LSL–Left Sacrolateral Position

LSM–Late Systolic Murmur

LSO–Lateral Superior Olive; Left Salpingo-oophorectomy

LSP–Left Sacroposterior Position

L/S Ratio–Lecithin/Sphingomyelin Ratio

LSS–Liver-Spleen Scan; Lumbosacral Spine

LST–Left Sacrotransverse

LSTL–Laparoscopic Tubal Ligation

LST Tract–Lateral Spinothalamic Tract

LSV–Left Subclavian Vein

LSWA–Large-Amplitude, Slow Wave Activity

LT–Left Thigh; Left Triceps; Leukotriene; Levin Tube; Levothyroxine; Low Transverse; Lumbar Traction

LTA–Leukotriene A

LTB–Laparoscopic Tubal Banding; Laryngotracheobronchitis; Leukotriene B

LTC–Leukotriene C; Long-Term Care

LTCS–Low Transverse Cesarean Section

LTG–Long-Term Goals

LTGA–Left Transposition of the Great Arteries

LTH–Lutotropic Hormone

LtH–Left-Handed

LTT–Lymphoblastic Transformation Test; Lymphocyte Transformation Test

L&U–Lower and Upper Extremities

LUE–Left Upper Extremity

LUL–Left Upper Lid; Left Upper Limb; Left Upper Lobe

LUO–Left Ureteral Orifice

LUOQ–Left Upper Outer Quadrant

LUSB–Left Upper Sternal Border

LV–Left Ventricle; Lung Volume

LVA–Left Ventricular Aneurysm
LVAD-Left Ventricular Assist Device
LVD–Left Ventricular Dysfunction
LVDP–Left Ventricular Diastolic Pressure
LVE–Left Ventricular Enlargement
LVED–Left Ventricular End–Diastolic
LVEDC–Left Ventricular End-Diastolic Circumference
LVEDP–Left Ventricular End-Diastolic Presure
LVEDV–Left Ventricular End-Diastolic Volume
LVEF–Left Ventriucular Ejection Fraction
LVEP–Left Ventricular End-Diastolic Pressure
LVEpi–Left Ventricular Epicardial Half
LVER–Liver Fraction(s) Elevated
LVET–Left Ventricular Ejection Time
LVETI–Left Ventricular Ejection Time Index
LVF–Left Ventricular Failure; Low-Voltage Fast; Low-Voltage Foci
LVFP–Left Ventricular Filling Pressure
L.V.G.–Left Ventrogluteal
LVH–Large Vessel Hematocrit; Left Ventricular Hypertrophy
LVI–Left Ventricular Insufficiency
LVID–Left Ventricular Internal Dimension
LVL–Left Vastus Lateralis
L.V.L.–Left Vastus Lateralis
LVLG–Left Ventrolateral Gluteal
LVMM–Left Ventricular Muscle Mass
LVO–Left Ventricular Overactivity
LVP–Large Volume Parenteral; Left Ventricular Pressure
LLVPW–Left Ventricular Posterior Wall
LVS–Left Ventricular Posterior Wall
LVS–Left Ventricular Strain
LVSP–Left Ventricular Systolic Pressure
LVSV-Left Ventricular Stroke Volume

LVSW–Left Ventricular Septal Wall; Left Ventricular Stroke Work

LVSWI–Left Ventricular Stroke Work Index

LVT–Left Ventricular Tension; Lysine Vasotonin

LVV–Left Ventricular Volume

LVVP–Chlorambucil, Vinblastine, Vincristine, and Prednisone

LVWI–Left Ventricular Work Index

LW–Lacerating Wound

LW–Lateral Wall; Lee-White

L & W–Living and Well

LWCT–Lachar-Wrobel Critical Items

LX–Local Irradiation

LXT–Left Exotropia

LYG–Lymphomatoid Granulomatosis

M

M–Malignant; Masculine; Massage; Medicine; Memory; Methotrexate; Microsporum; Molar; Multipara; Murmur; Muscle

MA–Mean Arterial; Menstrual Age; Mental Age; Mentum Anterior; Meter Angle; Mitomycin-C and Adriamycin; Mitral Annulus; Moderately Advanced; Muscle Activity

MAA–Monarticular Arthritis

MABOP–Nitrogen Mustard, Adriamycin, Bleomycin, Vincristine, and Prednisone

MABP–Mean Arterial Blood Pressure

MAC–Malignancy–Accociated Changes; Midarm Circumference; Minimun Aveolar Concentration;

Mitomycin-C, Adriamycin, and Cyclophophamide; Monitored Anesthesia Care

MACC–Methotrexate, Adriamycin, and CCNU; Methotrexate, Adriamycin, Cyclophosphamide

MAD–Methandriol; Methyl Lomustine and Adriamycin; Mind-Altering Drugs

MAE–Moves All Extremities; Multilingual Aphasia Examination

MAEEW–Moves All Extremities Equally Well

MAF–Minimum Audible Field

MAFAs–Movement-Associated Fetal Accelerations

MAHA–Macroangiopathic Hemolytic Anemia

MAIT–Methotrexate and Cytosine Arabinoside

MAL–Midaxillary Line

MAMA–Monoclonal Antimalignin Antibody

MAMC–Midarm Muscle Circumference

MAN–Magnocellular Nucleus

MAO–Medial Ankle Orthosis; Monoamine Oxidase

MAP–L-Phenylalanine Mustard, Adriamycin, and Prednisone; Mean Aortic Pressure; Mean Arterial Pressure; Megaloblastic Anemia of Pregnancy; Microlithiasis Alveolarum Pulmonum; Minimum Audible Pressure; Monophasic Action Potential; Muscle Action Potential; Muscle Aptitude Profile

MAPI–Millon Adolescent Personality Inventory

MARIA–Macroaggregated Radioiodinated Albumin

MAS–Manifest Anxiety Scale; Meconium Aspiration Syndrome; Mobile Arm Spport

MAT–Manual Arts Therapist; Miller-Abbott Tube; Multifocal Atrial Tachycardia

MAV–Minute Alveolar Volume

MB–Buccal Margin; Mesiobuccal

M-BACOD–Methotrexate, Citrovorum Factor, Bleomycin, Adriamycin, Cyclophosphamide, Vincristine, and Dexamethasone

MBC–Maximum Breathing Capacity

MBD–Methotrexate, Bleomycin, and Cis-Platinum; Minimal Brain Damage; Morquiio-Brailsford Disease

MBF–Myocardial Blood Flow

MBFLB–Monaural Bifrequency Loudness Balance

MBH–Medial Basla Hypothalamus

MBL–Medium Brown Loose; Menstrual Blood Loss

MBM–Mother's Breast Milk

MBO–Mesiobucco-Occlusal

MBP–MB Band Present; Mean Blood Pressure; Mesiobuccopulpul

MC–Mesenteric Collateral; Mesiocervical; Metacarpal; Metatarsocu-
    meiform; Mineralocorticoid; Miscarriage; Mitomycin; Mixed Cryo-
    globulinemia; Myocarditis

MCA–Main Coronary Artery; Major Coronary Arteries; Maternity
    Center Association; Middle Cerebral Aneurysm

McB–McBurney's Point

MCBP–Melphalan, Cyclophosphamide, Carmustine(BCNU) and
    Prednisone

MCC–Marked Contraction; Mean Corpuscular Hemoglobin
    Concentration; Midstream Clean-Catch

MCD–Medium Corpuscular Density; Medullary Cystic Disease;
    Metacarpal Cortical Density

MCDT–Mast Cell Degranulation Test

MCF–Medium Corpuscular Fragility; Myocardial Contractile Force

MCGN–Mixed Cryoglobulinemia Associated With Glomerulonephritis

MCH–Maternal and Child Health; Mean Cell Hemoglobin; Mean
    Corpuscular Hemoglobin

MCHC–Mean Corpuscular Hemoglobin Concentration

MCHL–Mean Corpuscular Hemoglobin

MCHS–Maternal and Child Health Service

MCI–Mean Cardiac Index

MCKD–Multicystic Kidney Disease

MCL–Medial Collateral Ligament; Midclavicular Line; Midcostal
    Line; Modified Chest Lead; Most Comfortable Level; Most Com-
    fortable Loudness

MCLNS–Mucocutaneous Lymph Node Syndrome

MCMAI–Millon Clinical Multi-Axial Inventory

MCP–Medical College of Pennsylvania; Melphalan, Cyclophosphamide, and Prednisone; Metacarpophalangeal

MCPH–Metacarpophalangeal

MCQ–Multiple Choice Question

MCS–Myocardial Contractile State

MCSA–Minimal Cross-Sectional Area

MCT–Mean Circulation Time; Mean Corpuscular Thickness; Medullary Cancer of the Thyroid; Multiple Compressed Tablet

MCTC–Metrizamide Computerized Tomographic Cisternography

MCTD–Mixed Connective Tissue Disease

MCV-Mean Cell Volume; Mean Corpuscular Volume

MD–Main Duct; Manic-Depression; Manic Depressive; Mantoux Diameter; Maternal Deprivation; Medium Dosage; Mental Deficienncy; Mesiodistal; Mitral Disease; Monocular Deprivation; Movement Disorder; Muscular Dystrophy Myocardial Damage; Myocardial Disease

MDA–Manual Dilation of the Anus; Motor Discriminative Acuity

MDAC–Multiplying Disital-to-Analog Converter

MDAP–Machover Draw-A-Person Test

MDBK–Madin-Darby Bovine Kidney

MC–Medial Dorsal Cutaneous Nerve

MDD–Major Depressive Disorder

MDF–Mean Dominant Frequency; Myocardial Depressant Factor

MDH–Medullary Dorsal Horn

MDHR–Maximum Determined Heart Rate

MDI–Manic-Depressive Illness; Metered Dose Inhaler; Multiple Daily Injection

MDII–Multiple Daily Insulin Injection

MDM–Mid-Diastolic Murmur

MDP–Mandibular Dysostosi and Peromelia; Manic-Depressive Psychosis; Maximum Deliverable Pressure

MDR–Mammalian Diving Response; Minimum Daily Requirement

MDS–Master of Dental Surgery; Maternal Deprivation Syndrome; Myocardial Depressant Substance

MDSO–Mentally Disordered Sex Offender

MDT–Mentodextra Transversa (Right Mentotransverse Position)

MDTA–McDonald Deep Test of Articulation

MDTP–Multidisciplinary Treatment Plan

MDUO–Myocardial Disease of Unknown Orgin

ME–Macular Edema; Medial Episiotomy; Median Eminence; Middle Ear

MEA–Multiple Endocrine Abnormalities; Multiple Endocrine Adenomatosis; Multiple Endocrine Adenopathy

MEA-I–Multiple Endocrine Adenomatosis Type I

MEC–Middle Ear Cells; Minimum Effective Concentration

MECG–Maternal Electrocardiogram

MED–Median Erythrocyte Diameter; Minimal Effective Dose; Minimal Erythema Dose

MEDAC–Multiple Endocrine Deficiency-Addison's Disease-Candidiasis

MEE–Middle Ear Effusion

MEF–Maximal Expiratory Flow; Middle Ear Fluid; Midexpiratory Flow

MEFR–Maximum Expiratory Flow Rate

MEFV–Maximum Expiratory Flow Volume

MEG–Magnetoencephalogram

MEN–Multiple Endocrine Neoplasia; Multiple Endocrinopathies

MEP–Mean Effective Pressure; Motor End-Plate; Multimodality Evoked Potential

MER–Mean Ejection Rate; Methanol-Extracted Residue of Bacille Calmette-Guerin; Myeloid-Erythrocyte Ratio

MES–Maintenance Electrolyte Solution; Maximum Electroshock Seizure

MET–Metabolic Equivalent of the Task; Metastasis; Midexpiratory Time

MF–Midcavity Forceps; Mitomycin-C and 5-Fluorouracil; Myocardial Fibrosis;

MFAT–Multifocal Atrial Tachycardia;

MFB–Metallic Foreign Body

MFCC–Marriage, Family, and Child Counselor

MFD–Mid-Forceps Delivery; Minimum Fatal Dose

MFEM–Maximal Forced Expiratory Maneuver

MFH–Membrane-Free Hemolysate

MFP–Myofascial Pain

MFR–Mid-Forceps Rotation; Mucus Flow Rate

MFT–Muscle Function Test

MFTVP–Motor-Free Test of Visual Perception

MFW–Multiple Fragment Wounds

MG–Marcus Gunn Pupil: Menopausal Gonadotropin; Mesiogingival; Michaelis-Gutmann; Muscle Group; Myasthenia Gravis

Mg–Magnesium (Chemical Symbol)

MGC–Minimal Glomerular Change

MGD–Mixed Gonadal Dysgenesis

MGM–Maternal Grandmother

MGN–Membranous Glomerulonephritis

MGP–Marginal Granulocyte Pool

MGR–Modified Gain Ratio; Murmurs, Gallops, or Rubs

MGUS–Monoclonal Gammopathies of Undetermined Significance

MGW–Magnesium Sulfate, Glycerine, Water

MH–Malignant Histiocytosis; Malignant Hyperpyrexia; Malignant Hyperthermia; Mammotropic Hormone; Medical History; Menstrual History; Mental Health

MHA–Microangiopathic Hemolytic Anemia

MHBSS–Modified Hank's Balanced Salt Solution

MHC–Major Histocompatibility Complex

MHD–Maintenance Hemodialysis; Mean Hemolytic Dose; Mental Health Department

MHDU–Medical Hemodialysis Unit

MHI–Mental Health Institute

MHN–Massive Hepatic Necrosis

MHR–Major Histocompatibility Region; Maximal Heart Rate; Methemoglobin Reductase

MHS–Major Histocomaptibility System; Malignant Hypothermia Susceptible; Maximum Histalog Stimulation

MHW–Medial Heel Wedge

MI–Menstrual Induction; Mental Institution; Mesioincisal; Mitral Incompetence; Mitral Insuffciency; Myocardial Infarction;

MIC–Maternal and Infant Care; Minimal Inhibitory Concentration; Minimal Isorrheic Concentration

MID–Maximum Inhibiting Duration; Mesioincisodistal; Minimal Infective Dose; Minimal Inhibiting Dose

MIF–Macrophage-Inhibiting Factor; Melanocyte-Stimulating Hormone Inhibiting Factor; Midinspiratory; Migration-Inhibitory Factor

MIFA–Mitomycin-C, 5-Fluorouracil, and Adriamycin

MIFR–Maximal Inspiratory Flow Rate

Mig–Membrane Immunoglobulin; Malaria Immunoglobulin; Measles Immunoglobin;

MIH–Melanocyte-Stimulating Hormone–Inhibitory Hormone; Migraine with Interparoxysmal Headache; Minimal Intermittent

MIN–Medial Interlaminar Nucleus

MIP–Maximum Inspiratory Pressure; Mean Intravascular Pressure; Middle Interphalangeal Joint

MIPS–Myocardial Isotopic Perfusion Scan

MIRD–Medical Internal Radiation Dose

MIRP–Myocardial Infarction Rehabilitation Program

MJL–Medial Joint Line

MKB–Megakaryoblast

ML–Lingual Margin; Malignant Lymphoma; Mesiolingual; Middle Lobe; Midline

MLA–Mesiolabial; Monocytic Leukemia, Acute

MLAP–Mean Left Atrial Pressure

MLaP–Mesiolabiopulpal

MLB–Monaural Loudness Balance

MLC–Minimal Lethal Concentration; Myelomonocytic Leukemia, Chronic

MLD–Median Lethal Dose; Metachromatic Leukodystrophy

MLF–Median Longitudinal Fasciculus

MLNS–Mucocutaneous Lymph Node Syndrome

MLO–Mesiolinguo-Occlusal

MLP–Mesiolinguopulpal

MLR–Mixed Lymphocyte Reaction

MLS–Mean Life Span; Myelomonocytic Leukemia, Subacute

MLT–Median Lethal Time; Mentolaeva Transversa

MM–Malignant Melanoma; Marshal Marchetti Operation; Medial Malleolus; Mixed Monitor; Mucous Membrane; Multiple Myeloma; Murmurs; Muscles; Muscularis Mucosa; Myeloid Metaplasia

MMC–Minimal Medullary Concentration; Mitomycin C

MMECT–Multiple Monitor Electroconvulsive Therapy

MMEF–Maximal Midexpiratory Flow

MMF–Maximum Midexpiratory Flow; Mean Maximum Flow

MMG–Mean Maternal Glucose

MMK–Marshall-Marchetti-Krantz

MMM–Myeloid Metaplasia with Myelofibrosis

MMOA–Maxillary Mandibular Odentectomy Alveolectomy

MMPI–McGill-Melzack Pain Index; Minnesota Multiphasic Personality Inventory

MMR–Mass Miniature Radiography; Maternal Mortality Rate; Measles, Mumps, and Rubella; Midline Malignant Reticulosis; Myocardial Metabolic Rate

MMT–Manual Muscle Test

MN–Mononuclear; Motor Neuron; Myoneural

Mn–Manganese (Chemical Symbol)

MNCL–Monoclonal Gammopathy Identified

MNCV–Motor Nerve Conduction Velocity

MND–Minimum Necrosing Dose; Motor Neuron Disease

MNG–Multinodular Goitor

MNJ–Myoneural Junction

MNL–Mononuclear Leukocytes

MNR–Marrow Neutrophil Reserve

MNTB–Medial Nucleus of the Trapezoid Body

MO–Manually Operated; Master of Obstetrics; Master of Osteopathy; Medial Oblique;

Mesio–Occlusal; Minute Output; No Evidence of Distal Metastasis

MOAD–Methotrexate, Vincristine, L-Asparaginase, and Dexamethasone

MOB–Nitrogen Mustard, Vincristine, and Bleomycin

MOC–Maximum Oxygen Consumption

MOCA–Methotrexate, Oncovin, Cytoxan, and Adriamycin

MOD–Maturity-Onset Diabetes; Mesio-Occlusodistal

MODM–Mature-Onset Diabetes Mellitus

MOF–Methotrexate, Oncovin, and 5-Fluorouracil

MOF-STREP–Methyl-CCNU(MeCCNU or Semustine) Vincristine, 5-Fluorouracil and Streptozocin

MOM–Milk of Magnesia

MOP–Nitrogen Mustard, Oncovin, and Prednisone; Nitrogen Mustard, Oncovin, and Procarbazine

MOP-BAP–Nitrogen Mustard, Vincristine, Procarbazine, Prednisone, Adriamycin, and Bleomycin

MOPP–Mechlorethamine, Oncovin, Procarbazine, and Prednisone; Methotrexate, Oncomycin, Prednisone, and Procarbazine; Mutine, Oncovin, Procarbazine, and Prednisone

MOPP-ABVD–Mechlorethamine, Vincristine, Procarbazine, Prednisone, Doxorubicin, Bleomycin, Vinblastine, and Dacarbazine

MOPP-LO BLEO–Mechlorethamine (mustargen), Oncovin, Procarbazine, Prednisone, and Bleomycin

MOPV–Monovalent Oral Poliovirus Vaccine

MOTT–Mycobacteria Other Than Tubercle

MOUS–Multiple Occurrences of Unexplained Symptoms

MP–Mean Pressure; Menstrual Period; Mentum Posterior; Mesiopulpal; Metacarpophalangeal; Metatarsophalangeal; Middle Phalanx; Monophosphate; Mouth Pressure; Mucopolysaccharide; Multiparous; Mycoplasmal Pneumonia; Myeloma Protein

MPA–Main Pulmonary Artery

MPAT–Mean Pulmonary Artery Pressure

MPB–Male Pattern Baldness

MPC–Maximum Permissible Concentration; Meperidine, Promethazine and Chlorpromazine; Myeloblastpromyelocyte Compartment

MPCU–Maximum Permissible Concentration of Unidentified Radionucleotides

MPD–Maximum Permissible Dose; Multiple Personality Disorder; Myofascial Pain Dysfunction

MPH–Methylphenidate

MPHR–Maximum Predicted Heart Rate

MPI–Maximum Permitted Intake; Maximum Point of Impulse; Multiphasic Personality Inventory; Myocardial Perfusion Imaging

MPJ–Metacarpophalangeal Joint; Metatarsophalangeal Joint

MPL–Maximum Permissible Level; Mesiopulpolingual

MPM–Malignant Papillary Mesothemioma; Multipurpose Meal

MPP–Massive Periretinal Proliferation; Maximum Perfusion Pressure

MPPT–Methylprednisolone Pulse Therapy

MPR–Marrow Production Rate

MPS–Michigan Picture Stories; Movement Produced Stimuli; Mucopolysaccharide; Multiphasic Screening

MPSMT–Merrill-Palmer Scale of Mental Tests

MPT–Morphine Provocative Test

MPV–Mean Platelet Volume; Metatarsus Primus Varus

MR–Magnetic Resonance; Measles-Rubella; Medial Rectus; Mental Retardation; Mitral Reflux; Mitral Regurgitation; Motivation Research; Muscle Relaxant

MRAP–Mean Right Atrial Pressure

MRBF–Mean Renal Blood Flow

MRD–Minimal Residual Disease; Minimal Reacting Dose; Minimum Reaction Dose

MRF–Melanocyte–Stimulating Hormone; Mesencephalic Reticular Formation; Midbrain Reticular Formation; Mitral Regurgitation Flow; Mullerian Regression Factor

MRG–Murmurs, Rubs, and Gallops

MRH–Melanocyte–Stimulating Hormone

MRI–Magnetic Resonance Imaging; Mental Research Institute; Moderate Renal Insufficiency

MRIF–Melanocyte-Stimulating Hormone

MRL–Minimum Response Level

MRO–Muscle Receptor Organ

MRR–Marrow Release Rate

MRS–Magnetic Resonance Spectroscopy

MRSH–Methicillin-Resistant Staphylococcus Aureus

MRT–Medical Records Technician; Muscle Response Test

MRU–Mass Radiographic Unit

MRV–Minute Respiratory Volume

MRVP–Mean Right Ventricular Pressure

MS–Maladjustment Score; Mental Status; Mentally Retarded; Mongolian Spot; Morphine Sulfate; Multiple Sclerosis; Muscle Shortening; Muscle Strength; Musculoskeletal

MSAF–Meconium Stained Amniotic Fluid

MSAFP–Maternal Serum Alpha Fetoprotein

MSB–Mid-Small Bowel

MSCA–McCarthy Scales of Children's Abilities

MSCE–Monitored Self-Care Evaluation

MSE–Mental Status Examination

MSER–Mean Systolic Ejection Rate

MSES–Medical School Environmental Stress

MSET–Multistage Exercise Test

MSG–Monosodium Glutamate

MSH–Medical Self-Help

MSK–Medullary Sponge Kidney; Musculoskeletal

MSKCC–Memorial Sloan-Kettering Cancer Center

MSL–Midsternal Line

MSLT–Multiple Sleep Latency Test

MSM–Medial Superior Olive

MSPGN–Mesangial Proliferative Glomerulonephritis

MSPS–Myocardial Stress Perfusion Scintigraphy

MSR–Muscle Stretch Reflexes

MSRPP–Multidimensional Scale for Rating Psychiatric Patients

MSS–Marital Satisfaction Scale; Mental Status Schedule; Minor Surgery Suite; Motion Sickness Susceptibility; Muscular Subaortic Stenosis

MST–Mean Survival Time

MSU–Maple Syrup Urine

MSV–Maximal Sustained Level of Ventilation

MSW–Multiple Stab Wound

MT–Malignant Teratoma; Malaria Therapy; Mammary Tumor; Metatarsal; Middle Turbinate; Muscles and Tendons; Muscle Therapy

MTA–Metatarsus Adductus

MTC–Medullary Thyroid Carcinoma; Mitomycin-C

MTCS–Madelian Thomas Completion Stories

MTD–Maximal Tolerated Dose

MTDDA–Minnesota Test for Differential Diagnosis of Aphasia

MTDT–Modified Tone Decay Test

MTF–Modulation Transfer Function

MTI–Malignant Teratoma Intermediate

MTJ–Midtarsal Joint

MTLP–Metabolic Toxemia of Late Pregnancy

MTP–Metatarsophalangeal Joint

MTR–Mass, Tenderness, Rebound; Mental Treatment Rules

MTS–Monosyllable, Trochee, Spondee Test

MTT–Malignant Trophoblastic Teratoma; Mean Transit Time

MTU–Malignant Teratoma Undifferentiated; Methylthiouracil

MTV–Metatarsus Varus

MUC–Maximum Urinary Concentration

MUGA–Multigated Angiogram; Multiple Gate Acquisition Analysis

MUGX–Multiple Gated Acquisition Exercise

MUO–Myocardiopathy of Unknown Origin

MUP–Motor Unit Potential

MURC–Measurable Undesirable Respiratory Contaminates

MUST–Medical Unit, Self-Contained, Transportable

MV–Minute Volume; Mitral Valve; Mixed Venous

MVA–Malignant Ventricular Arrhythmias; Mitral Valve Area; Motor Vehicle Accident

M-VAC–Methotrexate, Vinblastine, Doxorubicin and Cisplatin

MVB–Mixed Venous Blood

MVC–Maximum Vital Capacity; Maximal Voluntary Contraction; Myocardial Vascular Capacity

MVE–Mitral Valve Echo; Murray Valley Encephalitis

MVH–Methotrexate, VP-16 and Hexamethylmelamine

MVI–Multiple Vitamin Infusion

MVLS–Mandibular Vestibulolingual Sulcoplasty; Meecham Verbal Language Scale

MVP–Mitral Valve Prolapse

MVPD-26–Methotrexate, Citovorum Factor, VM-26, Procarbazine and Dexamethasone

MVPP–Mustine, Vinblastine, Procarbazine and Prednisone; Nitrogen Mustard, Vinblastine, Procarbazine and Prednisone

MVR–Massive Vitreous Retraction; Maximum Ventilation Rate; Mitral Valve Regurgitation; Mitral Valve Replacement

MVRI–Mixed Vaccine, Respiratory Infections

MVS–Mitral Valve Stenosis

MVT–Maximal Ventilation Time

MVV–Maximum Voluntary Ventilation; Maximum Voluntary Volume

MWS–Mikity-Wilson Syndrome

MYTGC–Miller-Yoder Test of Grammatical Comprehension

MZ–Mantle Zone

MZA–Monozygotic Twins Raised Apart

MZT–Monozygotic Twins Raised Together

N

N–Nasal; Nerve; Neuropathy; Nitrogen; Normal

NA–Narcotics Anonymous; Noradrenalin; Nucleus Ambiguus; Numerical Aperature; Nurse Anesthetist; Nursing Assistant

Na–Sodium (Chemical Symbol)

NAA–Neuron Activation Analysis; No Apparent Abnormalities

NAACLS–National Accrediting Agency for Clinical Laboratory Sciences

NABS–Normoactive Bowel Sounds

NAC–Nitrogen Mustard, Adriamycin and Lomustine

NAD–Nicotinamide Adenine Dinucleotide; Normal Axis Deviation; Nothing Abnormal Detected

NAF–National Amputation Foundation; National Ataxia Foundation

NAG–Narrow Angle Glaucoma

NAI–Nonaccidental Injury

NAP–Nasion Pogonion

NAR–Nasal Airway Resistance

NAS–Neonatal Abstinence Syndrome; No Added Salt

NB–Newborn; Needle Biopsy; Nitrous Oxide-Barbituate; No Bowel Movement; Normal Bowel Movement

NBA–Non-Weight-Bearing Ambulation

NBI–No Bone Injury

NBM–No Bowel Movement; Normal Bowel Movement; Nothing by Mouth

NBN–Narrow Band Nerve; Newborn Nursery

NBS–Normal Blood Serum; Normal Bowel Sounds

NBTE–Nonbacterial Thrombotic Endocarditis

NBTNF–Newborn, Term, Normal Female

NBTNM–Newborn, Term, Normal Male

NBW–Normal Birth Weight

NC–Nasal Cannula; Neural Crest; Neurocirculatory; Neurological Check; Noncompliance; Normocephalic

NCA–National Council on Aging; Neurocirculatory Asthenia

NCAT–Normocephalic and Atraumatic

NCB–No Code Blue

NCD–Normal Childhood Diseases; Not Considered Disabling

NCE–Nonconvulsive Epilepsy

NCF–Neutrophil Chemotactic Factor

NCI–Naphthalene, Creosote and Iodoform

NCJ–Needle Catheter Jejunostomy

NCL–Neuronal Ceroid Lipofuscinosis

NCMI–National Committee Against Mental Illness

NCNC–Normochromic, Normocytic

NCNCA–Normochromic, Normocytic Anemia

NCP–Nursing Care Plan

NCPE–Noncardiac Pulmonary Edema

NCPR–No Cardiopulmonary Resuscitation

NCS–Nerve Conduction Studies

NCT–Nerve Conduction Tests; Neural Crest Tumor

NCV–Nerve Conduction Velocity

ND–Nasal Deformity; Neonatal Death; Neoplastic Disease; Nervous Debility; Neurotic Depression; Newcastle Disease; Normal delivery; Normal Development; Nose Drops

N&D–Nodular and Diffuse

NDA–New Drug Application

NDC–National Drug Code

NDD–No Dialysis Days

NDDG–National Diabetes Data Group

NDE–Near Death Experience

NDF–New Dosage Form

NDI–Nephrogenic Diabetes Insipidus

NDP–Net Dietary Protein

NDT–Neurodevelopmental Treatment

NE–Nerve Ending; Nerve Excitability; Neurological Examination; Norepinephrine

NEC–Necrotizing Enterocolitis; Not Elsewhere Classifiable

NED–No Evidence of Disease; No Expiration Date

NEEP–Negative End-Expiratory Pressure

NEMD–Nonspecific Esophageal Motility Disorder

NEP–Negative Expiratory Pressure

NEPD–No Evidence of Pulmonary Disease

NET–Nasoendotracheal Tube

NEX–Nose to Ear to Xiphoid

NF–Nephritic Factor; Neurofibromatosis; Noise Factor; Normal Flow

NFAR–No Further Action Required

NFC–National Fertility Center

NFD–Neurofibrillary Degeneration

NFT–Neurofibrillary Tangle

NFTD–Normal Full-Term Delivery

NFTSD–Normal Full-Term Spontaneous Delivery

NFTT–Nonorganic Failure to Thrive

NFW–Nursed Fairly Well

NG–Nasogastric

NGC–Nucleus Reticularis Gigantocellularis

NGF–Nerve Growth Factor

NGR–Narrow Gauze Roll; Nasogastric Replacement

NGSA–Nerve Growth Stimulating Activity

NGU–Nongonococcal Urethritis

NH–Nodular Histiocytic; Nursing Home

NHA–National Hearing Association; Nonspecific Hepatocellular Abnormality

NHD–Normal Hair Distribution

NHL–Nodular Histiocytic Lymphoma; Non-Hodgkin's Lymphoma

NHP–Normal Human Pooled Plasma

NHS–Normal Human Serum

NHSM–No Hepatosplenomegaly

NI–Neurological Improvement; No Information; Noise Index

NIAL–Not in Active Labor

NIC–Neonatal Intensive Care; Noninvasive Carotid Study

NICE–Noninvasive Carotid Examination; Noninvasive Cerebrovascular Examination

NICU–Neonatal Intensive Care Unit; Neurological Intensive Care Unit

NIDD–Noninsulin-Dependent Diabetes

NIDDM–Noninsulin-Dependent Diabetes Mellitus

NIF–Negative Inspiratory Force

NIHL–Noise-Induced Hearing Loss

NINVS–Noninvasive Neurovascular Studies

NIP–Negative Inspiratory Pressure

NIPE–Noninvasive Peripheral Evaluation

NIT–National Intelligence Test

NJ–Nasojejunal

NKA–No Known Allergies

NKDA–No Known Drug Allergies

NKH–Nonketotic Hyperglycemia

NKHS–Nonketotic Hyperosmolar Syndrome

NL–Nasolacrimal; Nodular Lymphoma

NLA–National Leukemia Association; Neuroleptanalgesia

NLD–Nasolacrimal Duct; Nacrobiosis Lipoidica Diabeticorum

NLF–Nasolabial Fold

NLM–Noise Level Monitor

NLP–Neurolinguistic Programming; No Light Perception; Nodular Liquifying Panniculitis;

Normal Light Perception

NM–Neuromotor; Neuromuscular; Nodular Melanoma

NMD–Normal Muscle Development

NMF–National Migraine Foundation; Nonmigrating Fraction

NMJ–Neuromuscular Junction

NML–Nodular Mixed Lymphoma

NMP–Normal Menstrual Period

NMR–Nictitating Membrane Response; Nuclear Magnetic Resonance

NMS–Neuroleptic Malignant Syndrome; Neuromuscular Stimulator

NMT–Nuclear Medicine Technologist; Neuromuscular Tension

NMU–Neuromuscular Unit

NN–Neonatal; Nurse's Notes

NNA–Normochromic, Normocytic Anemia

NND–Neonatal Death

NNE–Neonatal Necrotizing Enterocolitis

NNI–Noise and Number Index

NNP–Neonatal Nurse Practitioner; Nerve Net Pulse

NNR–New and Nonofficial Remedies

NOMI–Nonocclusive Mesenteric Infarction

NP–Nasal Prongs; Nasopharyngeal; Neuropathology; Neurophysin; Neuropsychiatric; Normal Plasma; Normal Pressure; Not Pregnant; Nucleus Pulposus

NPA–Near-Point Accommodation

NPB–Nodal Premature Beat

NPC–Nasopharyngeal Carcinoma; Near Point of Convergence; Nodal Premature Contractions

NPCa–Nasopharyngeal Carcinoma

NPD–Niemann-Pick Disease

NPDL–Nodular Poorly Differentiated Lymphocytic

NPDR–Nonproliferative Diabetic Retinopathy

NPEV–Nonpolio Enterovirus

NPFT–Neurotic Personality Factor Test

NPH–Neutral Protamine Hagedorn; Normal Pressure Hydrocephalus

NPHS–Northwick Park Heart Study

NPI–Neuropsychiatric Institute

NPL–Nodular Poorly Differentiated Lymphoma

NPO–Non Per Os

NPT–Normal Pressure and Temperature

NR–No Resonse; Nodal Rhythm; Nonreactive; Nonrebreathing; Nonresponsive; Nutrition Ratio

NRA–Nucleus Raphe Alatus; Nucleus Retroambigualis

NRBS–Nonrebreathing System

NRC–Normal Retinal Correspondence

NREM–Nonrapid Eye Movement

NRH–Nodular Regenerative Hyperplasia

NRR–Note, Record, Report

NRT–Neuromuscular Re-Education Techniques

NS–Nephrosclerosis; Nephrotic Syndrome; Nervous System; Neurosecretory; Neurosurgery; Neurosyphilis; Normal saline; Nuclear Sclerosis; Nylon Suture

NSA–No Salt Added; No Significant Abnormality

NSAIA–Nonsteroidal Anti-Inflammatory Agent

NSAID–Nonsteroidal Anti-Inflammatory Drug

NSC–Neurosecretory Cells; No Significant Change

NSCLC–Non-Small-Cell Lung Cancer

NSD–No Significant Defect; Nominal Single Dose; Normal Spontaneous Delivery

NSDA–Nonsteroidal Dependent Asthmatic

NSF–Nodular Subepidermal Fibrosis

NSFTD–Normal Spontaneous Full-Term Delivery

NSG–Neurosecretory Granules

NSGCTT–Nonseminomatous Germ Cell Tumor of the Testis

NSI–Negative Self-Image

NSILA–Nonsuppressible Insulin-Like Activity

NSM–Neurosecretory Material

NSN–Nephrotoxic Serum Nephritis; Nicotine-Stimulated Neurophysin

NSND–Nonsymptomatic, Nondisabling; Nose Saline Nose Drops

NSPVT–Nonsustained Polymorphic Ventricular Tachycardia

NSQ–Neuroticism Scake Questionnaire

NSR–Nasoseptal Reconstruction; Normal Sinus Rhythm

NSRR–Normal Sinus Rate and Rhythm

NSS–Normal Saline Solution

NSSPAVAF–Normal Size, Shape and Position, Anteverted and Anteflexed

NSST–Nonspecific ST Segment Changes; Northwestern Syntax Screening Test

NST–Nonstress Test; Normal Shincter Tone

NSU–Nonspecific Urethritis

NSV–Nonspecific Vaginitis

NSVD–Normal Spontaneous Vaginal Delivery

NSVT–Nonsustained Ventricular Tachycardia

NT–Nasotracheal; Nephrostomy Tube; Normotensive

NTC–Neurotrauma Center

NTD–Neural Tube Defect

NTE–Not To Exceed

NTG–Nitroglycerin; Nontoxic Goiter

NTMNG–Nontoxic, Multinodular Goiter

NTMI–Nontransmural Myocardial Infarction

NTN–Nephrotoxic Nephritis

NTS–Nasotracheal Suction; Nucleus Tractus Solitarii

NUD–Nonulcer Dyspepsia

NUG–Necrotizing Ulcerative Gingivitis

NV–Neurovascular; Nonvaccinated; Nonvenereal

N&V–Nausea and Vomiting

NVA–Near Visual Acuity

NVD–Nausea, Vomiting and Diarrhea; Neck Vein Distention; Neo-vascularization of the Disc; Neurovesical Dysfunction; Nonvalvular Disease

NVE–Neovascular Edema

NVG–Neovascular Glaucoma

NVSS–Normal Variant Short Stature

NVT–Nerve, Vein and Tendon

NWB–Non-Weight Bearing

O

O–Obstetrics; Occiput; Occlusal; Oral; Orbit; Oxygen;

OA–Occiptial Artery; Occiput Anterior; Oral Alimentation; Osteoarthritis

O & A–Observation and Assessment

OAD–Obstructive Airway Disease

OAP–Oncovin, ARA-C, Prednisone; Ophthalmic Artery Pressure; Osteoarthropathy; Oxygen at Atmospheric Pressure

OAP-BLEO–Oncovin, ARA-C, Prednisone, Bleomycin

OAV–Oculoauriculovertebral Dysplasia

OAWO–Opening Abductory Wedge Osteotomy

OB–Obstetrics; Occult Bleeding

OBD–Organic Brain Disease

OB-GYN–Obstetrics and Gynecology

OBN–Occult Blood Negative

OBP–Occult Blood Positive; Ova, Blood, and Parasites

OBS–Organic Brain Syndrome

OC–Obstetrical Conjugate; Occlusocervical; Only Child; Oral Contraceptive

OCA–Oculocutaneous Albinism; Oncovin, Cyclophosphatmide, and Adriamycin

OCCC–Open Chest Cardiac Compression

OCCM–Open Chest Cardiac Message

OCD–Osteochondritis Dissecans; Ovarian Cholesterol Depletion Test

OCG–Oral Cholecystogram

OCN–Oculomotor Nucleus;

OCP–Oral Contraceptive Pill; Ova, Cysts, Parasites

OCS–Open Canalicular System

OCT–Oxytocin Challenge Test

OCV–Ordinary Conversational Voice

OD–Occupational Disease; Ocular Density; Oculus Dexter; Overdose

ODA–Occipito-Dextra Anterior

ODAP–Oncovin, Diahydrogalactitol, Adriamycin, and Cis-Platinum

ODB–Opiate-Directed Behavior

ODD–Oculodentodigital Dysplasia

ODP–Occipito-Dextra Posterior

ODQ–Opponens Digiti Quinti

OE–On Examination; Otitis Externa

O & E–Observation and Evaluation

OEE–Outer Enamel Epithelium

OEM–Open-End Marriage

OER–Osmotic Erythrocyte Enrichment; Oxygen Enhancement Ratio

OF–Occipitofrontal; Orbitofrontal; Osteitis Fibrosa

OFC–Occipital-Frontal Circumference

OFD–Object-Film Distance

OG–Occlusogingival; Optic Ganglion; Orogastric;

OGD–Old Granulomatus Disease

OGF–Orogastric Feeding; Ovarian Growth Factor

OGS–Oxogenic Steroid

OGTT–Oral Glucose Tolerance Test

OH–Hydroxycorticosteroid; Occupational Health; Open Heart; Oral Hygiene; Osteopathic Hospital

OHC–Occupational Health Center

OHD–Organic Heart Disease

OHF–Omsk Hemorrhagic Fever

OHG–Oral Hypoglycemic

OHI–Ocular Hypertension Indicator

OHN–Occupation Health Nurse

OHP–Oxygen High Pressure; Oxygen Under Hyperbaric Pressure

OHRR–Open Heart Recovery Room

OI–Orgasmic Impairment; Orientation Inventory; Osteogensis Imperfecta; Oxygen Income; Oxygen Index; Oxygen Intact

OIP–Organizing Interstitial Pneumonia

OIRD–Object-to-Image Receptor Distance

OIT–Organic Integrity Test

OKN–Optokinetic Nystagmus

OLA–Occipitolaeva Anterior

OLH–Ovine Lactogenic Hormone

OLP–Abnormal Llipoprotein; Occipitolaeva Posterior

OLT–Occipitolaeva Transversa

OM–Obtuse Marginal; Occipitomental; Ochsner-Mahorner; Osteomalacia; Osteomyelitis; Otitis Media; Ovulation Method

OMAD–Oncovin, Methotrexate, Citrovorum Factor, Adriamycin, and Actinomycin-D

OMCA–Otitis Media, Catarrhal, Acute

OMD–Ocular Muscular Dystrophy

OMI–Old Myocardial Infarction

OMPA–Otitis Media, Purulent, Acute

OMR–Operative Mortality Rate

OMSC–Otitis Media, Secretory, Chronic; Otitis Media, Suppurative, Chronic

ON–Optic Nerve; Ortho-Novum; Orthopedic Nurse

ONC–Over-the-Needle Catherter

OND–Other Neurological Disorders

ONP–Operating Nursing Procedure

ONTR–Orders Not To Resuscitate

OP–Occiput Posterior; Opening Pressure; Operative Procedure; Ophthalmology; Oropharynx; Osmotic Pressure; Osteoporosis; Other Than Psychotic

O & P–Ova and Parasites

OPAL–Oncovin, Adriamycin, L-Asparaginase, and Prednisone

OPC–Oxypneumocardiogram

OPCA–Olivopontocerebellar Atrophy

OPD–Optical Path Difference; Otopalatodigital

OPE–Orbiting Primate Experiment

OPG–Ocular Plethysmography

OPA/CPA–Oculoplethysmography/Carotid Phonoangiography

OPLL–Ossification of Posterior Longitudinal Ligament

OPM–Occult Primary Malignancy

OP–Occiput Posterior Position; Oncovin, Procarbazine, and Prednisone; Oxygen Partial Pressure

OPPG–Oculopneumoplethysmography

OPV–Oral Poliovirus

OQSMAT–Otis Quick Scoring Mental Abilities Tests

OR–Oil Retention; Open Reduction; Operating Room; Own Recognizance

ORIF–Open Reduction and Internal Fixation

ORN–Operating Room Nurse; Orthopedic Nurse

ORS–Oral Surgeon; Orthopedic Surgeon

ORT–Operating Room Technician

OS–By Mouth; Oculus Sinister; Opening Snap; Oral Surgery; Orthopedic Surgery; Osgood-Schlatter; Osteogenic Sarcoma; Osteosarcoma; Osteosclerosis

OSA–Obstructive Sleep Apnea

OSM–Oxygen Saturation Meter

OSMED–Otospondylomegaepiphyseal Dystrophy

OST–Object Sorting Test

OT–Objective Test; Occlusion Time; Occupational Therapist; Old Tuberculin; Olfactory Threshold; Otis Test

OTC–Over-The-Counter; Oxytetracycline

OTD–Organ Tolerance Dose

OU–Oculi Unitas; Oculus Uterque

OURQ–Outer Upper Right Quadrant

OV–Ovary; Overventilation

OVD–Occlusal Vertical Dimension

OVLT–Organum Vasculosum of the Lamina Terminalis

OW–Open Wedge; Out-of–Wedlock

P

P–Parity; Partial Pressure; Partial Tension; Passive; Percussion; Perforation; Perfusionist; Porphyrin; Premolar; Pressure; Primipara; Prolactin; Protein; Pulse; Pupil

PA–Paralysis Agitans; Paranoia; Periapical; Pernicious Anemia; Phakic-Aphakic; Pituitary-Adrenal; Plasma Aldosterone; Plasminogen Activator; Polyarteritis; Posterior-Anterior; Primary Amenorrhea; Primary Anemia; Prolonged Action Pulmonary Artery; Pulmonary Atresia; Pulpoaxial

P & A–Percussion and Auscultation

PAB–Premature Atrial Beat;

PABA–Para-Aminobenzoic Acid

PAC–Papular Acrodermatitis of Childhood; Parent-Adult-Child; Premature Artial Contraction

PACE–Cis-Platinum, Adriamycin, Cyclophosphamide, and Vindesine; Personalized Aerobics for Cardiovascular Enhancement

PACP–Pulmonary Artery Counter-Pulsation

PACS–Picture Archiving and Communications

PAD–Percutaneous Abscess Drainage; Percutaneous Automated Diskectomy; Peripheral Arterial Disease; Phenacetin, Aspirin, Desoxyephedrine; Primary Affective Disorder; Psychoaffective Disorder; Pusatile Assist Device

PADA–Pulmonary Artery Diastolic Pressure

PAF–Paroxysmal Atrial Fibrillation; Platelet Activating Factor; Platelet Aggregation Factor; Pulmonary Arteriovenous Fistula

PA & F–Percussion, Auscultation, and Fremitus

PAFIB–Paroxysmal Atrial Fibrillation

PAG–Pariaqueductal Grey Matter

PAGE–Program for Automated Gated Evaluation

PAH–Para-Aminohippurate; Pulmonary Artery Hypertension; Pulmonary Artery Hypotension

PAIgG–Platelet-Associated Immunoglobulin G

PAIVS–Pulmonary Atresia with Intact Ventricular Septum

PAL–Posterior Axillary Line

PALN–Para-Aortic Lymph Node

PALS–Paired Associate Learning Subtest

PAM–Potential Acuity Meter; Primary Amoebic Meningoencephalititis; Pulmonary Alveolar Macrophages

PAN–Periarteritis Nodosa; Periodic Alternating Nystagmus; Polyarteritis Nodosa; Positional Alcohol Nystagmus

PAOD–Peripheral Arterial Occlusive Disease

PAOP–Pulmonary Artery Occlusion Pressure

PAP–Papanicolaou; Peak Airway Pressure; Positive Airway Pressure; Primary Atypical Pneumonia; Pulmonary Alveolar Proteinosis; Pulmonary Artery Pressure

PAPVC–Partial Anomalous Pulmonary Venous Connection

PAPVR–Partial Anomalous Pulmonary Venous Return

PAR–Platelet Aggregate Ratio; Postanesthetic Recovery; Probable Allergic Rhinitis; Pulmonary Arteriolar Resistance

PARU–Postanesthetic Recovery Unit

PAS–Peripheral Anterior Synechia; Progressive Accumulated Stress; Pulmonary Artery Stenosis

PAT–Paroxysmal Atrial Tachycardia; Pregnancy At Term; Psychoacoustic Testing

PATCO–Prednisone, Vincristine, Thioguanine, Cytosine Arabinoside, and Cyclophosphamide

PATE–Pulmonary Artery Thromboembolectomy

PAW–Peak Airway Pressure; Pulmonary Artery Wedge

PAWP–Pulmonary Arterial Wedge Pressure

PB–Pressure Breathing

PBA–Percutaneous Bladder Aspiration; Pressure Breathing Assister; Pulbobuccoaxial

PBC–Peripheral Blood Cells; Point of Basal Convergence; Primary Biliary Cirrhosis

PBF–Pulmonary Blood Flow

PBI–Partial Bony Impaction; Penile-Brachial Index

PBLI–Premature Birth, Live Infant

PBN–Paralytic Brachial Neuritis; Polymyxin B Sulfate, Bacitracin, and Neomycin

PBP–Peak Blood Pressure

PBSP–Prognostically Bad Signs During Pregnancy

PBV–Predicted Blood Volume; Pulmonary Blood Volume

PC–Packed Cells; Plasmacytoma; Platelet Concentrate; Pneumotaxic Center; Portacaval; Postcoital; Posterior Circumflex; Posterior

Chamber; Precordium; Premature Contraction; Psychodevelopment
Checklist; Pubococcygeus; Pulmonary Capillary; Pulmonic Closure

PCA–Passive Cutaneous Anaphylaxis; Patient–Controlled Analgesia;
Percutanous Carotid Arteriogram; Porous-Coated Anatomic; Posterior
Cerebral Artery; Posterior Communicating Artery

PCB–Paracervical Block; Postcoital Bleeding

PCC–Pheochromocytoma; Premature Chromosome Condensation;
Prothrombin-Complex Concentration

PCCU–Post Coronary Care Unit

PCD–Polycystic Disease; Posterior Corneal Deposits; Pulmonary
Clearance Delay

PCDUS–Plasma Cell Dyscrasia of Unknown Significance

PCE–Pulmocutaneous Exchange

PCEN–Paracentesis Fluid

PCF–Pharygoconjunctival Fever; Posterior Cranial Fossa

PCG–Paracervical Ganglion; Phoncardiogram; Pubococcygeus

PCH–Paroxysmal Cold Hemoglobinuria

PCI–Prophylactic Cranial Irradiation

PCIOL–Posterior Chamber Intraocular Lens

PCKD–Polycystic Kidney Disease

PCL–Persistent Corpus Luteum; Posterior Chamber Lens; Posterior
Cruciate Ligamen

PCN–Penicillin; Percutaneous Nephrostomy

PCO–Patient Complains Of

PCOD–Polycystic Ovary Disease

PCON–Platelet Concentration

PCP–Peripheral Coronary Pressure; Pneumocystic Pneumonia; Pneu-
mocystis Carinii Pneumonia Principal Care Provider; Pulmonary
Capillary Pressure

PCS–Palliative Care Service; Portacabal Shunt; Primary Cancer Site

PCSM–Percutaneous Stone Manipulation

PCT–Plasmacrit Test; Plasmacytoma; Porcine Calcitonin; Porphyria Cutenea Tarda; Portacaval Transpostition; Postcoital Test; Prothrombin Consumption Time; Proximal Convoluted Tubule

PCU–Pain Control Unit

PCV–Packed Cell Volume; Parietal Cell Vagotomy; Polycythemia Vera; Procarbazine, Lomustine(CCNU), and Vincristine

PCW–Pulmonary Capillary Wedge

PCWP–Pulmonary Capillary Wedge Pressure

PCXR–Portable Chest Xray

PD–Papilla Diameter; Paralyzing Dose; Parkinsonism Dementia; Parkinson's Disease; Pars Distalis; Patent Ductus; Percutaneous Drain; Peritoneal Dialysis; Plasma Defect; Poorly Differentiated; Postnasal Drainage; Potential Difference; Pressor Dose; Psychopathic Deviate; Psychotic Depression; Pulmonary Disease; Pulpodistal; Pupillary Distance

PDA–Patent Ductus Arteriosus; Pediatric Allergy; Posterior Descending Artery; Principal Diagonal Artery

PDC–Pediatric Cardiology; Psychodevelopment Checklist

PD&C–Postural Drainage and Clapping

PDE–Paroxysmal Dyspnea on Exertion; Pulsed Doppler Echocardiography

PDFC–Premature Dead Female Child

PDFG–Platelet-Derived Growth Factor

PDH–Past Dental History

PDI–Psychomotor Development Index

PDL–Poorly Differentiated Lymphocytic

PDLL–Poorly Differentiated Lymphocytic Lymphoma

PDMC–Premature Dead Male Child

PD&P–Postural Drainage and Percussion

PDR–Pediatric Radiology; Proliferative Diabetic Retinopathy

PDS–Pain Dysfunction Syndrome; Paroxysmal Depolarizing Shift; Pediatric Surgery; Peritoneal Dialysis System

PDGXT–Predischarge Graded Exercise Test

PDU–Pulsed Doppler Ultrasonography

PDWHF–Platelet-Derived Wound Healing Factor

PE–Pericardial Effusion; Phakoemulsification; Pharyngoesophageal; Pleural Effusion; Pneumatic Equalization; Pressure Equalization; Pulmonary Edema; Pulmonary Embolism

PEARL–Pupils Equal and React to Light

PEEP–Positive End-Expiratory Pressure

PEF–Peak Expiratory Flow; Psychiatric Evaluation Form

PEFR–Peak Expiratory Flow Rate

PEFSR–Partial Expiratory Flow-Static Recoil Curve

PEFV–Partial Expiratory Flow Volume

PEG–Percutaneous EndoscopicGastrostomy; Pneumoenxephalogram

PEM–Prescription-Event Monitoring; Pulmonary Embolus

PEMF–Pulsing Electromagnetic Field

PEN–Parenteral and Enteral Nutrition; Penicillin

PENG–Photoelectric Mystagmography

PEO–Progressive External Ophthalmoplegia

PEP–Cyclophosphamide, VM-26, and Prednisolone; Pre-Ejection Period; Psychiatric Evaluation Profile

PEPI–Pre-Ejection Period Index

PEEP–Positive Expiratory Pressure Plateau

PERK–Prospective Evaluation of Radial Keratotomy

PERLA–Pupils Equal and Reactive to Light and Accommodation

PERR–Pattern-Evoked Retinal Response

PERRLA–Pupils Equal, Round, and Reactive to Light and Accommodation

PET–Parent Effectiveness Training; Positron-Emission Tomography; Pre-Eclamptic Toxemia; Pressure Equalization Tubes; Psychiatry Emergency Team

PET Scan–Positron Emission Tomographic Scan

PF–Peak Factor; Peak Flow; Peritoneal Fluid; Personality Factor; Phenylalanine and Methotrexate; Picture Frustration; Plantar Flexion; Platelet Factor; Posterior Fontanelle; Pulmonary Factor; Purkinje Fibers

PFA–Profunda Femoris Artery

PFB–Pseudofolliculitis Barbae

PFC–Pelvic Flexion Contracture; Persistent Fetal Circulation

PFEAAC–Posterior Fossa Extra-Axial Arachnoid

PFFD–Proximal Femoral Focal Deficiency

PFM–Peak Flow Meter

PFO–Patent Foramen Ovale

PFP–Platelet-Free Plasma

PFQ–Personality Factor Questionaire

PFR–Parotid Flow Rate; Peak Flow Rate; Pulmonary Flow Rate

PFS–Pulmonary Function Score

PFT–Pancreatic Function Test; Parafascicular Thalamotomy; Penylalanine Mustard(Melphalan) , Fluorouracil, Tamoxifen; Posterior Fossa Tumor; Pulmonary Function Tests

PG–Pituitary Gonadotropin; Plasma Glucose; Pregnandiol Glucuronide; Prostaglandin; Pyoderma Gangrenosum

PGA–Prostaglandin A

PGE–Platelet Granule Extract

PGF–Paternal Grandfather

PGH–Pituitary Growth Hormone; Plasma Growth Hormone

PGI–Potassium, Glucose, and Insulin

PGL–Persistent Generalized Lymphadenopathy

PGN–Proliferative Glomerulonephritis

PGO–Ponto-Geniculo-Occipital

PGP–Post-Gamma Proteinuria

PGR–Psychogalvanic Response

PGTR–Plasma Glucose Tolerance Rate

PGU–Postgonoccal Urethritis

PH–Past History; Porta Hepatis; Prostatic Hypertrophy; Pulmonary Hypertension; Purpura Hyperglobinemia

PHA–Peripheral Hyperalimentation; Pulse Height Analyzer

PHC–Premolar Aplasia, Hyperhidrosis, and Premature Cavities; Primary Hepatic Carcinoma; Primary Hepatocelluar Carcomona; Proliferative Helper Cells

PHF–Paired Helical Filaments

PHFG–Primary Human Fetal Glia

PHG–Phosphatidylglycerol

PHH–Posthemorrhagic Hydrocephalus

PHIM–Posthypoxic Insertion Myoclonus

PHN–Postherpetic Neuralgia

PHP–Primary Hyperparathyroidism; Pseudohypoparathyroidism

PHPV–Persistent Hyperplastic Primary Vitreous

PHR–Peak Heart Rate

PHS–Posthypnotic Suggestion

PHTS–Psychiatric Home Treatment Service

PHV–Persistent Hypertrophic Vitreous

PI–Pacing Impulse; Paranoid Ideation; Performance Intensity; Peripheral Iridectomy; Personality Inventory; Physically Impaired; Pneumatosis Intestinalis; Porch Index; Pregnancy Induced; Preinduction; Primary Infarction; Psychiatric Institute; Pulmonary Incompetence; Pulmonary Infarction; Pulmonary Insufficiency

PIAT–Peabody Individual Achievement Test

PICA–Porch Index of Communicative Ability; Posterior Inferior Cerebellar Artery; Posterior Inferior Communicating Artery; Posterior Internal Cerebral Artery

PICU–Pediatric Intensive Care Unit; Pulmonary Intensive Care Unit

PID–Pelvic Inflammatory Disease; Prolapsed Intervertebral Disc

PIDRA–Portable Insulin Dosage-Regulating Apparatus

PIE–Preimplantation Embryo; Pulmonary Infiltrate With Eosinophilia; Pulmonary Interstitial Edema

PIF–Peak Inspiratory Flow; Prolactin Inhibiting Factor

PIFR–Peak Inspiratory Flow Rate

PIFT–Platelet Immunofluorescence Test

PIH–Pregnancy-Induced Hypertension; Prolactin Release-Inhibiting Hormone

PIP–6-Mercaptopurine, Vincristine, Methotrexate, and Citroborum Factor; Peak Inspiratory Pressure; Proximal Interphalangeal; Psychotic Impatient Profile

PIR–Postinhibitory Rebound

PIT–Patellar Inhibition Test; Picture Identification Test; Plasma Iron Turnover

PITR–Plasma Iron Turnover Rate

PIVD–Protruded Intervertebral Disc

PJB–Premature Junctional Beat

PJC–Premature Junctional Contraction;

PJS–Peutz-Jeghers Syndrome

PK–Penetrating Deratoplasty; Prausnits-Kunstner; Psychokinesis

PKD–Polycystic Kidney Disease

PKU–Phenylketonuria

PKV–Killed Poliomyelitis Vaccine

PL–Perception of Light; Peroneus Longus; Placental Lactogen; Pulpolingual

PLA–Pulpolabila; Pulpolinguoaxial

PLD–Platelet Defect; Potentially Lethal Damage; Pregnancy, Labor, and Delivery

PLDD–Poorly Differentiated Lymphoma, Diffuse

PLE–Protein-Losing Enteropathy

PLED–Periodic Lateralized Epileptiform Discharge

PLEVA–Pityriasis Lichenoides et Varioliformis Acuta

PLF–Perilmyphatic Fistula

PLFC–Premature Living Female Child

PLGV–Psittacosis-Lymphogranuloma Venereum

PLH–Paroxysmal Localized Hyperhidrosis

PLIF–Postlumbar Interbody Fusion

PLL–Peripheral Light Loss; Prolymphocytic Leukemia

PLMC–Premature Living Male Child

PLN–Pelvic Lymph Node; Popliteal Lymph Node; Posterior Lip Nerve

PLR–Pronation/Lateral Rotation

PLS–Preschool Language Scale; Primary Lateral Sclerosis; Prostaglandin-Like Substance

PLT–Primed Lymphocyte Typing; Psittacosis–Lymphogranuloma Venereump Trachoma;

PLV–Live Poliomyelitis Vaccine; Panleukopenia Virus; Phenylalanine-Lysine-Vasopressin; Posterior Left Ventricle

PM–Pacemaker; Poliomyelitis; Polymorphonuclear; Polymyositis; Postmenopausal; Premolar; Presystolic Murmur; Preventive Medicine; Primary Motivation; Prostatic Message; Pulpomesial

PMA–Papillary, Marginal, Attached; Premenstrual Asthma; Prevalence of Gingivitis; Prinzmetal's Angina; Progressive Muscular Atrophy

PMB–Cis-Platinum, Methotrexate, and Bleomycin; Postmenopausal Bleeding

PMC–Pseudomembranous Colitis

PMD–Primary Myocardial Disease; Progressive Muscular Dystrophy

PME–Polymorphonuclear Eosinophils; Postmenopausal Estrogen

PMF–L-Phenylalanine Mustard, 5-Fluorouracil, and Methotrexate; Progressive Massive Fibrosis

PMH–Past Medical History

PMHR–Predicted Maximal Heart Rate

PMI–Past Medical Illness; Patient Medication Instructions; Point of Maximal Impulse Posterior Myocardial Infarction

PML–Polymorphonuclear Leukocytes; Posterior Mitral Leaflet; Progressive Multifocal Leukoencephalopathy

PMMA–Polymethyl Methacrylate

PMN–Polymorphonuclear Leukocyte; Polymorphonuclear Neutrophil

PMNG–Polymorphonuclear Granulocytes

PMNR–Periadentitis Mucosa Necrotica Recurrens

PMO–Postmenopausal Osteoporosis

PMP–Pain Management Program; Past Menstrual Period; Persistent Mentoposterior; Previous Menstrual Period

PMR–Perinatal Mortality Rate; Physical Medicine and Rehabilitation; Polymorphic Reticulosis; Polymyalgia Rheumatica; Posteromedial Release

PMS–Phenazine Methosulfate; Postmenopausal Syndrome; Premenstrual Symdrome; Pureed, Mechanical , Soft

PMT–Porteus Maze Test; Premenstrual Tension

PMTS–Premenstrual Tension Syndrome;

PMTT–Pulmonary Mean Transit Time

PMV–Prolapse of Mitral Valve

PN–Parenteral Nutrition; Perceived Noise; Percussion Note; Periarteritis Nodasa; Peripheral Nerve; Polyarteritis Nodosa; Positional Nystagmus; Postnasal; Postnatal; Psychiatry-Neurology; Pyelonephritis

PNAS–Prudent No Salt Added

PNB–Premature Nodal Beat; Prostatic Needle Biopsy

PNC–Penicillin; Peripheral Nerve Conduction; Pneumotaxic Center; Premature Nodal Contraction; Prenatal Care; Prenodal Contraction

PND–Paroxysmal Nocturnal Dyspnea; Postnasal Drainage

PNF–Proprioceptive Neuromuscular Facilitation

PNH–Paroxysmal Nocturnal Hemoglobinuria

PNI–Peripheral Nerve Injury; Postnatal Infection; Prognostic Nutrition Index

PNMG–Persistent Neonatal Myasthenia Gravis

PNP–Peripheral Neuropathy; Progressive Nuclear Palsy

PNPR–Positive-Negative Pressure Respiration

PNS–Parasympathetic Nervous System; Partial Nonprogressing Stroke; Peripheral Nerve Stimulator

PNSS–Pediatric Nutrition Surveillance System

PNT–Percutaneous Nephrostomy Tube

PNV–Prenatal Vitamins

Pnx–Pneumothorax

PO–Partial Pressure of Oxygen; Parieto-Occipital; Postoperative

P&O–Parasites and Ova

POA–Pancreatic Oncofetal Antigen; Phalangeal Osteoarthritis; Preoptic
Area; Primary Optic Atrophy

POACH–Prednisone, Oncovin, Cytosine Arabinoside, Cyclophosphamide and Adriamycin

POAG–Primary Open-Angle Glaucoma

POB–Place of Birth; Prevention of Blindness

POC–Postoperative Care; Products of Conception

POCA–Adriamycin, Prednisone, Cytosine Arabinoside and Oncovin

POCC–Procarbazine, Oncovin, CCNU and Cyclophosphamide

POD–Place of Death; Postoperative Day

POE–Postoperative Endophthalmitis

POEMS–Plasma Cell Dyscrasia with Polyneuropathy, Organomegaly,
Endocrinopathy, Monclonal Protein, Skin Changes

POET–Pulse Oximeter/ End Tidal

POHI–Physically or Otherwise Health-Impaired

POI–Personal Orientation Inventory

POL–Premature Onset of Labor

POLE–Prednisone, Oncovin and L-Asparaginase

POMP–Prednisone, Vincristine, Methotrexate and 6-Mercaptopurine

POMR–Problem-Oriented Medical Records

POP–Persistent Occiputoposterior; Plasma Oncotic Pressure; Plaster of
Paris; Popliteal

PORP–Partial Ossicular Replacement Prosthesis

PORT–Postoperative Respiratory Therapy

POS–Parosteal Osteosarcoma; Polycystic Ovarian Syndrome

POSS–Proximal Over-Shoulder Strap

POSTS–Positive Occipital Sharp Transients of Sleep

POU–Placenta, Ovary and Uterus

POW–Powassan Encephalitis

PP–Pancreatic Polypeptide; Parodoxical Pulse; Partial Pressure; Pallagra Preventative; Perfusion Pressure; Permanent Partial; Pink Puffers; Pinpoint; Pin Prick; Placental Protein; Planned Parenthood; Posterior Pituitary; Post Partum; Postprandial; Prothrombin-Proconvertin; Protoporphyrin; Proximal Phalanx; Pulse Pressure

PPA–Phenylpropanolamine; Postpartum Amenorrhea

PP&A–Percussion, Palpation and Auscultation

PPB–Platalet-Poor Blood; Positive Pressure Breathing

PPBS–Postprandial Blood Sugar

PPC–Proximal Palmar Crease

PPCA–Plasma Prothrombin Conversion Accelerator

PPD–Packs Per Day; Percussion and Postural Drainage; Permanent Partial Disability; Posterior Polymorphous Dystrophy; Postpartum Day; Progressive Perceptive Deafness; Purified Protein Derivative

PPF–Pellagra Preventative Factor; Phagocytosis Promoting Factor

PPG–Pediatric Pneumogram; Photoplethysmography

PPGF–Polypeptide Growth Factor

PPH–Postpartum Hemorrhage; Primary Pulmonary Hypertension

PPHN–Persistent Pulmonary Hypertension of the Neonate

PPHP–Pseudo-Pseudohypoparathyroidism

PPI–Patient Package Insert

PPL–Pars Planus Lensectomy

PPLO–Permanent Pacemaker; Posterior Papillary Muscle

PPMD–Posterior Polymorphous Dystrophy of the Cornea

PPN–Peripheral Parenteral Nutrition

PPNA–Peak Phrenic Nerve Activity

PPP–Passage, Power and Passenger; Platelet-Poor Plasma; Postpartum Psychosis

PPPBL–Peripheral Pulses Palpable, Both Legs

PPPG–Postprandial Plasma Glucose

PPROM–Prolonged Premature Rupture of Membranes

PPRWP–Poor Precordial R-Wave Progression

PPS–Personal Preference Scale; Polyvalance Pneumococcal Polysa-ccharides; Postpartum Sterilization; Postperfusion Syndrome; Post-pump Syndrome; Prausnitz-Kustner Sclerosis

PPSB–Prothrombin, Proconvertin, Stuart Factor, Antihemophilic B Factor

PPTL–Postpartum Tubal Ligation

PPV–Positive-Pressure Ventilation

PPVT–Peabody Picture Vocabulary Test

PQ–Pronator Quadratus

PR–Parallax and Refraction; Partial Remission; Pelvic Rock; Perfusion Rate; Peripheral Resistance; Posterior Repair; Predicted Rate; Progesterone Receptor; Pulmonic Regurgitation; Pulse Rate

P&R–Pelvic and Rectal; Pulse and Respiration

PRA–Progesterone Receptor Assay

PRB–Personal Reaction Blank; Prosthetics Research Board

PRBC–Packed Red Blood Cells

PRBV–Placental Residual Blood Volume

PRCA–Pure Red Cell Agenesis; Pure Red Cell Aplasia

PRD–Postradiation Dysplasia

PRE–Physical Reconditioning Exercises

PREs–Progressive Resistive Exercises

PRF–Pontine Reticular Formation

PRFM–Prolonged Rupture of Fetal Membranes

PRG–Phleborrheogram

PRHBF–Peak Reactive Hyperemia Blood Flow

PRI–P-R Interval

PRIME–Procarbazine, Ifosfamide and Methotrexate

PRM–Premature Rupture of Membranes

prn–Pro Re Nata (As Needed)

PROM–Passive Range of Motion; Premature Rupture of Membranes; Prolonged Rupture of Membranes

PRO-MACE–Adriamycin, Cyclophosphamide, Methotrexate, Prednisone and VP-16

PROVIMI–Proteins, Vitamins and Minerals

PRP–Panretinal Photocoagulation; Pityrisis Rubra Pilaris; Platelet-Rich Plasma; Progressive Rubella Panencephalitis; Proliferative Retinopathy Photocoagulation; Psychotic Reaction

Profile; Pulse Repetition Frequency

PRRE–Pupils Round, Regular, Equal

PRS–Personality Rating Scale

PRSs–Positive Rolandic Spikes

PRU–Peripheral Resistance Unit

PRV–Polycythemia Vera

PRVEP–Pattern Reversal Visual Evoked Potentials

PRW–Polymerized Ragweed

PRWP–Poor R-Wave Progression

PS–Paradoxical Sleep; Pathological Stage; Pediatric Surgery; Perceptual Speed Test; Performance Status; Performing Scale; Plastic Surgery; Point of Symmetry; Porter-Silber; Psychiatric; Pulmonary Stenosis; Pyloric Stenosis

P&S–Pain and Suffering; Paracentesis and Suction

PSA–Prolonged Sleep Apnea; Prostate-Specific Antigen

PsA–Psoriatic Arthritis

PSC–Posterior Subcapsular Cataract; Primary Sclerosing Cholangitis; Pulse Synchronized Contractions

PSCE–Presurgical Coagulation Evaluation

PSCP–Posterior Subcapsular Cataractous Plaque

PSE–Point of Subjective Equality; Portal Systemic Encephalopathy

PSF–Posterior Spinal Fusion; Pseudosarcomatous Fasciitis

PSG–Peak Systolic Gradient; Phosphate-Saline-Glucose; Polysomnogram; Presystolic Gallop

PSGN–Poststreptococcal Glomerulonephritis

PSH–Postspinal Headache

PSI–Posterior Sagittal Index; Problem Solving Information; Psychosomatic Solving Information; Psychosomatic Inventory

PSIL–Preferred-Frequency Speech Interference Level

PSIS–Posterior Sacroiliac Spine; Posterior Superior Iliac Spine

PSL–Parasternal Line

PSM–Panasystolic Murmur; Presystolic Murmur

PSMA–Progressive Spinal Muscular Atrophy

PSP–Pace-Setting Potential; Pancreatic Spasmolytic Peptide; Parathyroid Secretory Protein; Positive Spike Pattern; Postsynaptic Potential; Progressive Supranuclear Palsy; Pseudo-pregnancy

PSR–Extrahepatic Portal Systemic Resistance; Pain Sensitivity Range

PSRLOW–Premature Spontaneous Rupture of Lung of Waters

PSS–Physiological Saline Solution; Progressive Systemic Sclerosis

PST–Paroxysmal Supraventricular Tachycardia; Pascal-Suttle Test; Penicillin, Streptomycin and Tetracycline; Poststimulus Time

PSV–Pressure Support Ventilation; Psychological, Social and Vocational

PSVT–Paroxysmal Supraventricular Tachycardia

PT–Parathyroid; Paroxysmal Tachycardia; Permanent and Total; Pharmacy and Therapeutics; Physical Training; Pneumothorax; Posterior Tibial; Pronator Teres; Prothrombin Time; Pulmonary Tuberculosis; Pyramidal Tract

PTA–Percutaneous Transluminal Angioplasty; Persistent Truncus Arteriosus; Plasma Thromboplastin Antecedent; Posterior Tibial; Postraumatic Amnesia; Pretreatment Anxiety; Prior to Admission

PTB–Patellar Tendon Bearing; Prior to Birth

PTBD–Percutaneous Transhepatic Biliary Drainage

PTBD-EF–Percutaneous Transhepatic Biliary Drainage-Enteric Feeding

PTC–Percutaneous Transhepatic Cholangiogram; Pheochromocytoma, Thyroid Carcinoma; Plasma Thromboplastin Component; Posterior Trebeculae Carneae; Prothrombin Complex

PTCA–Percutaneous Transluminal Coronary Angioplasty

PTD–Prior to Discharge; Permanent Total Disability

PTE–Parathyroid Extract; Pretibial Edema; Proximal Tibial Epiphysis; Pulmonary Thrombo-embolism

PTF–Plasma Thromboplastin Factor; Proximal Tubule Fluid

PTH–Parathyroid Hormone; Phenylthiohydantoin; Posttransfusion Hepatitis

PTL–Perinatal Telencephalic Leukoencephalopathy; Preterm Labor

PTLD–Prescribed Tumor Lethal Dose

PTM–Posttetanic Potentiation; Posttransfusion Mononucleosis

PTMDF–Pupil, Tension, Media, Disk, Fundus

PTP–Posterior Tibial Pulse Pulse; Posttetanic Potentiation

PTPM–Posttraumatic Progressive Myelopathy

PTPN–Peripheral Vein Total Parenteral Nutrition

PTR–Peripheral Total Resistance; Perlsucht-Tuberculin Rest

PTSD–Posttraumatic Stress Disorder

PTT–Partial Thromboplastin Time; Pateller Tendon Transfer; Pulmonary Transit Time

PTX–Parathyroidectomy; Pneumothorax

PU–Peptic Ulcer; Per Urethra; Pregnancy Urine; Prostatic Urethra

PUBS–Percutaneous Umbilical Blood Sampling

PUD–Peptic Ulcer Disease; Pulmonary Disease

PUE–Pyrexia of Unknown Etiology

PUH–Pregnancy Urine Hormone

PUL–Percutaneous Ultrasonic Lithotripsy

PULSES Profile–Physical Condition, Upper Extremity Function, Lower Extremity Function, Sensory and Communication Abilities, Excretory Control, Social Support

PUNL–Percutaneous Ultrasonic Nephrolithotripsy

PUO–Pyrexia of Undetermined Origin

PUPPP–Pruritic Urticarial Papillary Plaques of Pregnancy

PUVA–Psoralens and Ultraviolet A

PV–Paraventricular; Peripheral Vascular; Peripheral Vein; Plasma Volume; Poliomyelitis Vaccine; Polycythemia Vera; Portal Vein; Postvoiding; Pressure/Volume; Pulmonary Vein; Pulmonic Valve

P&V–Percuss and Vibrate; Pyloroplasty and Vagotomy

PVAS–Postvasectomy

PVB–Cis-Platinum, Vinblastine and Bleomycin; Premature Ventricular Beat

PVBS–Possible Vertebral-Basilar System

PVC–Postvoiding Cystogram; Premature Ventricular Contraction; Primary Visual Cortex; Pulmonary Venous Congestion

PVD–Parent Very Disturbed; Percussion, Vibration and Drainage; Peripheral Vascular Disease; Posterior Vitreous Detachment; Pulmonary Vascular Disease

PVE–Perivenous Encephalomyelitis; Premature Ventricular Extrasystole; Prosthetic Valve Endocarditis

PVEP–Pattern Visual Evoked Potential

PVF–Peripheral Visual Field; Portal Venous Flow; Posterior Vitreous Face

PVH–Preventricular Hemorrhage

PVI–Peripheral Vascular Insufficiency; Personal Values Inventory

PVM–Proteins, Vitamins and Minerals

PVNS–Pigmented Villonodular Synovitis

PVO–Peripheral Vascular Occlusion; Pulmonary Venous Occlusion

PVOD–Peripheral Vascular Occlusive Disease; Pulmonary Venous Obstructive Disease

PVP–Peripheral Vein Plasma; Peripheral Venous Pressure; Portal Vein Pressure

PVR–Peripheral Vascular Resistance; Postvoid Residual; Proliferative Vitreoretinopathy; Pulmonary Vascular Resistance; Pulse-Volume Recording

PVS–Percussion, Vibration and Suction; Peripheral Vascular Surgery; Peritoneovenous Shunt; Persistent Vegetative State; Premature Ventricular Systole; Pulmonic Valve Stenosis

PVT–Paroxysmal Ventricular Tachycardia; Portal Vein Thrombosis; Pressure, Volume and Temperature

PW–Plantar Wart; Posterior Wall

PWB–Partial Weight-Bearing

PWC–Peak Work Capacity

PWI–Posterior Wall Infarct

PWLV–Posterior Wall of Left Ventricle

PXE–Pseudoxanthoma Elasticum

PYA–Psychoanalysis

PZ-CCK–Pancreozymin-Cholecystokinin

PZI–Protamine Zinc Insulin

PZP–Pregnancy Zone Protein

Q

Q–Blood Volume; Cardiac Output; Perfusion; Quantity; Quinidine; Volume of Blood

QA–Quality Assurance

QAM–Quaque Ante Meridiem

QAP–Quinidine, Atabrine and Pamaquine

QAR–Quality Assurance Reagent; Quantitative Autoradiographic

QB–Quantitative Battery; Whole Blood

QBC–Quality Buffy Coat; Quantitative Buffy Coat

QBV–Whole Blood Volume

QC–Quality Control; Quinine-Colchicine

Qc–Pulmonary Capillary Blood Flow

QCA–Quantitative Coronary Angiography

QCT–Quantitative Computerized Tomography

QEE–Quadriceps Extension Exercise
QF–Quality Factor
QH–Quaque Hora (Every Hour)
QHS–Quaque Hora Somni (At Bedtime)
QID–Quater in Die (Four Times a Day)
QJ–Quadriceps Jerk
QMT–Quantitative Muscle Testing
QO–Oxygen Consumption
QOD–Quaque Other Die (Every Other Day)
QOH–Quaque Other Hora (Every Other Hour)
QON–Quaque Other Nocte (Every Other Night)
QP–Quadrant Pain; Qualified Psychiatrist
Qp–Pulmonary Blood Flow
QPC–Quadrigeminal Plate Cistern
Qpc–Pulmonary Capillary Blood Flow
QPEEG–Quantitative Pharmaco-Electroencephalography
QPM–Quaque Post Meridiem (Every Night)
QPT–Quick Prothrombin Time
QPVT–Quick Picture Vocabulary Test
QQH–Quaque Quarta Hora (Every Four Hours)
QR–Quantum Rectum (Quantity is Correct); Quick Recovery
QS–Every Shift; Quiet Sleep; Quantum Sufficit (As Much as Will Suffice)
Qs/Qt–Intrapulmonary Shunt Ratio; Right-to-Left Shunt Ratio
QSS–Quantitative Sacroiliac Scintigraphy
Q's Sign–Quant's Sign
Q-S Test–Queckenstedt-Stookey Test
QT–Blood Volume Quantity Per Unit of Time; Cardiac Output; Queckenstedt's Test; Quick Test
QUART–Quadrantectomy, Axillary Dissection and Radiotherapy
QUICHA–Quantitative Inhalation Challenge Apparatus
QV–Quantum Volueris (As Much as You Wish)

QW–Quality of Working Life

R

R–Behnken's Unit; Radiographer; Rectal; Respiration; Right Eye; Rorschach Test

RA–Radioactive; Radium (Chemical Symbol); Ragweed Antigen; Raynaud's Phenomenon; Renal Artery; Residual Air; Rheumatoid Arthritis; Right Atrium; Rokintansky-Aschoff

RAA–Renin-Angiotensin-Aldosterone; Right Atrial Appendage

RAB Diet–Rice, Applesauce and Banana Diet

RABG–Room Air Blood Gases

RAC–Right Atrial Catheter

RAD–Reactive Airway Disease; Right Anterior Descending; Right Axis Deviation; Roentgen Administered Dose

RADISH–Rheumatoid Arthritis Diffuse Idiopathic Skeletal Hyperostosis

RADP–Right Acromiodorsoposterior

RAE–Right Atrial Enlargement

RAEB–Refractory Anemia, Erythroblastic; Refractory Anemia with Excess of Blastocytes

RAEM–Refractory Anemia with Excess Myeloblasts

RAF–Rheumatoid Arthritis Factor

RAG–Room Air Gas

Ragg–Rheumatoid Agglutinator

RAIU–Radioactive Iodine Uptake

RAM–Rapid Alternating Movements

RAQ–Right Anterior Oblique; Right Anterior Occipital

RAP–Renal Artery Pressure; Right Atrial Pressure

RAPD–Relative Afferent Pupillary Defect

RAR–Right Arm Recumbent

RAS–Renal Artery Stenosis; Reticular Activating System; Rheumatoid Arthritis Serum

RAST–Radioallergosorbent Test

RAT–Repeat Action Tablet; Right Anterior Thigh

RAW–Airway Resistance

RAZ–Razoxane

RB–Respiratory Bronchiole; Retrobulbar; Right Bronchus; Right Buttock

R&B–Right and Below

RBA–Rescue Breathing Apparatus; Right Brachial Artery

RBB–Right Breast Biopsy; Right Bundle Branch

RBBB–Right Bundle Branch Block

RBC–Red Blood Cell

RBCD–Right Border of Cardiac Dullness

RBCM–Red Blood Cell Mass

RBCV–Red Blood Cell Volume

RBD–Right Border of Dullness

RBE–Relative Biological Effectiveness

RBF–Renal Blood Flow

RBL–Reid's Base Line

RBN–Retrobulbar Neuritis

RBOW–Ruptured Bag of Water

RBP–Resting Blood Pressure

RBS–Random Blood Smear; Random Blood Sugar

RBTC–Rational Behavior Therapy Center

RBV–Right Brachial Vein

RC–Reaction Center; Respiration Center; Respiratory Ceases; Retention Catheter; Retrograde Cystogram; Root Canal

RCA–Radionuclide Cerebral Angiogram; Red Cell Agglutination; Right Coronary Artery

RCBV–Regional Cerebral Blood Volume

RCC–Radiochemical Center; Rape Crisis Center; Red Cell Count; Renal Cell Carcinoma; Routine Coronary Care

RCD–Relative Cardiac Dullness

RCFS–Reticulocyte Cell-Free System

RCG–Radiocardiography

RCI–Respiratory Control Index

RCM–Red Cell Mass; Right Costal Margin

RCR–Respiratory Control Ratio

RCS–Reticulum Cell Sarcoma

RCT–Root Canal Therapy; Rorschach Content Test

RCU–Respiratory Care Unit

RD–Reynaud's Disease; Registered Dietician; Renal Disease; Research Department; Respiratory Disease; Retinal Detachment; Reye's Disease; Right Deltoid; Right Dorsal; Ruptured Disc

RDA–Recommended Daily Allowance; Right Dorsoanterior Position

RDI–Rupture-Delivery Interval

RDOD–Retinal Detachment, Oculus Dexter

RDOS–Retinal Detachment, Oculus Sinister

RDP–Right Dorsoposterior

RDPE–Reticular Degeneration of the Pigment Epithelium

RDS–Respiratory Distress Syndrome

RDT–Regular Dialysis Treatment; Retinal Damage Threshold

RDVT–Recurrent Deep Vein Thrombosis

RDW–Red Cell Distribution Width

RE–Radium Emanation; Rectal Examination; Regional Enteritis; Reticuloendothelial; Right Eye

REA–Renal Anastomosis

REB–Roentgen-Equivalent Biological

R-EBD-HS–Recessive-Epidermolysis Bulbosa Dystrophica-Hallopeau Siemens

RECG–Radioelectrocardiogram

REE–Rapid Extinction Effect

REEG–Radioelectroencephalograph

REEL–Receptive-Expressive Emergent Language Scale

REF–Renal Erythropoietic Factor

REFMS–Recreation and Education for Multiple Sclerosis Victims

REG–Radiation Exposure Guide; Radioencephalogram

REM–Rapid Eye Movement; Roentgen Equivalent Man

REMAB–Radiation Equivalent Maniken Absorption

REO–Respiratory and Enteric Orphan

REP–Retrograde Pyelogram; Roentgen Equivalent Physical

RER–Renal Excretion Rate; Respiratory Exchange Ratio

RF–Radial Fibers; Radiofrequency; Receptive Field; Renal Failure; Respiratory Failure; Rheumatic Fever; Root Canal, Filling of

RFA–Right Femoral Artery; Right Frontoanterior Position

RFB–Retained Foreign Body

RFL–Right Frontolateral Position

RLFA–Rheumatoid-Factor-Like Activity

RFP–Right Frontoposterior Position

RFS–Rapid Frozen Section

RFT–Right Frontotransverse Position

RFV–Right Femoral Vein

RG–Retrograde; Right Gluteal

RGAS–Retained Gastric Antrum Syndrome

RGC–Retinal Ganglial Cells

RGM–Right Gluteus Maximus

RGP–Retrograde Pyelogram

RH–Radiological Health; Reactive Hyperemia; Releasing Hormone; Rheumatic; Right Hand; Right Hyperphoria; Room Humidifier

RH–Rhodium (Chemical Symbol)

RHB–Raise Head of Bed; Right Heart Bypass

RHBF–Resin Hemoperfusion Column; Respirations Have Ceased; Right Hypochondrium

RHD–Relative Hepatic Dullness; Rheumatic Heart Disease

RHF–Right Heart Failure

RHL–Right Hemisphere Lesion; Right Hepatic Lobe

RHLN–Right Hilar Lymph Node
RHM–Roentgen per Hour at one Meter
RHR–Resting Heart Rate
RHS–Right-Hand Side
RHT–Right Hypertropia
RI–Radiation Intensity; Refractive Index; Regional Ileitis; Regular Insulin; Remission Induction; Respiratory Illness; Retroactive Inhibition; Right Iliac Crest
RIA–Radioimmune Assay
RIAST–Reitan Indiana Aphasic Screening Test
RIC–Right Iliac Crest; Right Internal Carotid
RICM–Right Intercostal Margin
RICS–Right Intercostal Space
RID–Reversible Intravascular Device
RIF–Rifampicin; Right Iliac Fossa; Right Internal Fixation
RIFA–Radio Iodinated Fatty Acid
RIHSA–Radioactive Iodinated Human Serum Albumin
RIM–Radioisotope Medicine
RIMA–Right Internal Mammary Anastomosis
RIND–Resolving Ischemic Neurological Defect
RIO–Right Inferior Oblique
RIOJ–Recurrent Intrahepatic Obstructive Jaundice
RIP–Rapid Infusion Pump
RIR–Right Iliac Region; Right Inferior Rectus
RISA–Radioactive Iodinated Serum Albumin
RIT–Rorschach Inkblot Test
RIV–Ramus Interventicularis; Right Innominate Vein
FJ–Radial Jerk; Robert Jones Dressing
RK–Radial Keratoplasty; Radial Keratotomy;Right Kidney
RKG–Radiocardiogram
RKH–Rokitansky-Kuster-Hauser Syndrome
RKW–Renal Potassium Wasting

RKY–Roentgenkymography

RL–Radiation Laboratory; Reduction Level; Reticular Lamina; Right Lateral; Right Leg; Right Lower; Right Ling

RLBCD–Right Lower Border of Cardiac Dullnes

RLC–Residual Lung Capacity

RLD–Related Living Donor; Ruptured Lumbar Disk

RLE–Right Lower Extremity

RLF–Retained Lung Fluid; Retrolental Fibroplasia; Right Lateral Femoral

RLL–Right Lower Limb

RLN–Recurrent Laryngeal Nerve; Regional Lymph Node

RLND–Regional Lymph Node Dissection

RLP–Radiation-Leukemia-Protection

RLQ–Right Lower Quadrant

RLR–Right Lateral Rectus

RLSO–Unit Released By Blood Bank

RLT–Right Lateral Thigh

RM–Radical Mastectomy; Range of Motion; Raven's Matrices; Red Marrow; Repetitions Maximum; Respiratory Movement

RMA–Relative Medullary Area; Right Mentoanterior

RMBF–Regional Myocardial Blood Flow

RMCA–Right Main Coronary Artery; Right Middle Cerebral Artery

RMCAT–Right Middle Cerebral Artery Thrombosis

RMCL–Right Midclavicular Line

RMCT–Rat Mast Cell Technique

RMD–Rapid Movement Disorder; Retromanubrial Dullness; Right Manubrial Dullness

RME–Right Mediolateral Episiotomy

RMEE–Right Middle Ear Exploration

RML–Right Mediolateral; Right Middle Lobe

RMP–Rifampicin; Right Mentoposterior Position

RMR–Right Medial Rectus

RMS–Rectal Morphine Sulfate; Rehabilitation Medicine Service; Respiratory Muscle Strength

RMT–Relative Medullary Thickness; Retromolar Trigone; Right Mentotransverse Position

RMV–Respiratory Minute Volume

RN–Radionuclide; Red Nucleus

Rn–Radon (Chemical Symbol)

RNA–Radionuclide Angiography; Rough, Noncapsulated Avirulent

RND–Radical Neck Dissection

RNEF–Resting (Radio-) Nuclide Ejection Fraction

RO–Reverse Osmosis

ROA–Right Occipitoanterior Position

ROAD–Reversible Obstructive Airway Disease

ROAP–Rubidazone, Oncovin(Vincristine), Cytosine Arabinoside, and Prednisone

ROI–Region of Interest

ROL–Right Occipitolateral Position

ROM–Range of Motion; Rupture of Membranes

ROP–Retinopathy of Prematurity; Right Occipitoposterior Position

RO & R–Rey Osterreigh and Recall Test

ROSC–Restoration of Spontaneous Circulation

ROT–Remedial Occupational Therapy; Right Occipitotransverse Postition

RP–Pulse Rate Index; Radial Pulse; Raynaud's Phenomenon; Refractory Period; Respiratory Rate; Resting Potential; Resting Pressure; Rest Pain; Retinitis Pigmentosa; Retinitis Proliferans; Retrograde Pyelography; Retroperitoneal

RPA–Reverse Passive Anaphylaxis; Right Pulmonary Artery

RPC–Reticularis Pontis Caudalis

RPCF–Reiter Protein Complement Fixation

RPCU–Retropubic Cystourethropexy

RPD–Removable Partial Denture

RPE–Retinal Pigment Epithelial
RPF–Relaxed Pelvic Floor; Renal Plasma Flow
RPG–Radiation Protection Guide; Retrograde Pyelogram
RPGN–Rapidly Progressive Glomerulonephritis
RPI–Reticulocyte Production Index
RPICCE–Round Pupil Intracapsular Cataract Extraction
RPLAD–Retroperitoneal Lymphoadenectomy
RPM–Rapid Processing Mode; Raven's Progressive Matrices
RPN–Renal Papillary Necrosis
RPO–Right Posterior Oblique
RPP–Retropubic Prosatectomy
RPPI–Role Perception Picture Inventory
RPPR–Red Cell Precursor Production Rate
RPR–Rapid Plasma Reagin
RPS–Renal Pressor Substance
RPU–Retropubic Urethropexy
RPV–Right Pulmonary Vein
RQ–Respiratory Quotient
RR–Radiation Response; Recovery Room; Red Reflex; Regular Respirations; Regular Rhythm; Respiratory Rate; Response Rate; Riva-Rocci (Sphygmomanometer)
RRAM–Repetitive and Rapid Alternating Movements
RRE–Round, Regular, and Equal
RREF–Resting Radionuclide Ejection Fraction
RR-HPO–Rapid Recompensation –High Pressure Oxygen
RRP–Relative Refractory Period
RS–Rauwolfia Serpentina; Recipient's Serum; Rectal Sinus; Reinforcing Stimulus; Reiter's Syndrome; Renal Specialist; Respiratory Syncytial; Reye's Syndrome; Rheumatoid Spondylitis; Right Sacrum
RSA–Reticulum Cell Sarcoma; Right Sacroanterior; Right Subclavian Artery
RSB–Right Sternal Border

RSC–Rested-Stated Contraction; Right-Side Colon Cancer

RScA–Right Scapuloanterior Position

RSCT–Rach Sentence Completion Test; Rotter Sentence Completion Test

RSD–Reflex Sympathetic Dystrophy

RSDS–Reflex-Sympathetic Dystrophy Syndrome

RSE–Reverse Sutured Eye; Right Sternal Edge

RSES–Reitan Strength of Grip

RSIVP–Rapid Sequence Intravenous Pyelogram

RSL–Right Sacrolateral Position

RSO–Right Salpingo-Oophorectomy

RSP–Rhinoseptoplasty; Right Sacroposterior Position

RSS–Russian Spring–Summer Encephalitis

RST–Reagin Screen Test; Right Sacrotransverse Position

RSV–Respiratory Syncytial Virus; Right Subclavian Vein; Rous Sarcoma Virus

RSW–Right-Sided Weakness

RT–Radiology Technologist; Radiotherpay; Reading Test; Recreational Therapy; Renal Transplant;

Right Thigh; Right Triceps

RTA–Renal Tubular Acidosis

RTF–Respiratory Tract Fluid

RTI–Respiratory Tract Infection

RTKP–Radiothermokeratoplasty

RTL–Reactive to Light

rTNM–Retreatment Tumor, Nodes, and Metastasis

RTOG–Radiation Therapy Oncology Group

RTPA–Recombinant Tissue-Type Plasminogen Activator

rtPA–Recombinant Tissue-Type Plasminogen Activator

RTR–Red Blood Cell Turnover Rate

RTRR–Return to Recovery Room

RTS–Real Time Scan

RTT–Radiation Therapy Technologist; Respiratory Therapy Technician
RU–Radioactive Uptake; Rectourethral; Retrograde Urogram; Right Upper
RUA–Routine Urinalysis
RUBIDIC–Rubidazone and Dacarbazine
RUG–Retrograde Ureterogram
RUL–Right Upper Lid; Right Upper Lung
RUO–Right Upper Outer Quandrant; Right Ureteral Orifice
RUOQ–Right Upper Outer Quadrant
RUQ–Right Upper Quadrant
RURTI–Recurrent Upper Respiratory Tract Infections
RUSB–Right Upper Sternal Border
RV–Rectovaginal Residual Volume; Respiratory Volume; Right Ventricle; Rubella Vaccine
RVA–Renal Vascular Resistance
RVD–Relative Vertebral Density
RVDV–Right Ventricular Diastolic Volume
RVE–Right Ventricular Enlargement
RVEDP–Right Ventricular End-Diastolic Volume
RVEF–Right Ventricular Ejection Fraction
RVESP–Right Ventricular End-Systolic Pressure
RVESV–Right Ventricular End-Systolic Volume
RVET–Right Ventricular Ejection Time
RVG–Radionuclide Ventriculography; Right Ventrogluteal; Right Visceral Ganglion
RVH–Renovascular Hypertension; Right Ventricular Hypertrophy
RVID–Right Ventricular Internal Dimension
FVL–Right Vastus Lateralis
RVLG–Right Ventrolateral Gluteal
RVO–Relaxed Vaginal Outlet; Retinal Vein Occlusion; Right Ventricular Overactivity
RVOA–Right Ventricular Overactivity

RVOT–Right Ventricular Outflow Tract
RVP–Renal Venous Plasma
RVR–Rapid Ventricular Response; Renal Vascular Resistance
RVRA–Renal Vein Renin Assay
RVS–Reported Visual Sensation
RVSW–Right Ventricular Stroke Work
RVSWI–Right Ventricular Stroke Work Index
RVT–Renal Vein Thrombosis
RX–Prescription; Treatment
RXLI–Recessive X-Linked Ichthyosis
RXT–Right Exotropia

S

S–Sacral; Saline; Salmonella; Semilente; Septum; Staphylococcus; Stimulus; Subcutaneous; Suction; Surgeon; Surgery;
SA–Sacrum Anterior; Salicylic Acid; Sarcoma; Schizophrenics Anonymous; Secondary Amenorrhea; Secondary Anemia; Self-Analysis; Sinoatrial; Sinus Arrhythmia; Staphylococcus aureus; Sternal Angle; Stokes-Adams; Surface Area; Sustained Action
SAB–Significant Asymptomatic Bacteriuria; Spontaneous Abortion; Subarachnoid Bleed; Subarachnoid Block
SABP–Spontaneous Acute Bacterial Peritonitis
SAC–Short–Arm Cast
SACD–Subacute Combined Degeneration
SACE–Serum Angiotensin Converting Enzyme
SACH–Solid, Ankle, Cushion Heel
SAD–Seasonal Affective Disorder; Small Airway Disease; Source to Axis Distance; Sugar, Acetone, Diacetic Acid Test
SADS–Seasonal Affective Disorder Syndrome
SAF–Self-Articulating Femoral

SAH–Subarachnoid Hemorrhage; Systemic Arterial Hypertension

SAM–Self-Administered Medication; Sex Arousal Mechanism; Streptozocin, Adriamycin and Methyl-CCNU; Systolic Anterior Motion

SAN–Sinoatrial Node

SANC–Short-Arm Navicular Cast

SAP–Serum Alkaline Phosphatase; Staphylococcus Aureus Proteus; Systemic Arterial Pressure

SAPD–Self-Administration of Psychotropic Drugs

SAQ–Short-Arc Quadriceps

SAR–Sexual Attitude Reassessment; Structure Activity Relationship

SARA–System for Anesthetic and Respiratory Analysis

SAS–Short-Arm Splint; Sklar Aphasia Scale; Sleep Apnea Syndrome; Sterile Aqueous Suspension; Supravalvular Aortic Stenosis

SAT–Senior Apperception Test; Speech Awareness Threshold; Subacute Thyroiditis; Systematized Assertive Therapy

SATL–Surgical Achilles Tendon Lengthening

SAVD–Spontaneous Assisted Vaginal Delivery

SB–Sengstaken-Blakemore Tube; Shortness of Breath; Sinus Bradycardia; Small Bowel; Spina Bifida; Stanford-Binet; Sternal Border; Stillbirth

SBC–Standard Bicarbonate

SBD–Straight Bag Drainage

SBE–Self-Breast Examination; Subacute Bacterial Endocarditis; Shortness of Breath on Exertion

SBEP–Somatosensory Brain Stem Evoked Potential

SBF–Slanchnic Blood Flow

SBFT–Small-Bowel Follow-Through

SBGM–Self Blood Glucose Monitoring

SBI–Systemic Bacterial Infection

SBIS–Stanford-Binet Intelligence Scale

SBMPL–Simultaneous Binaural Mid Plane Localization Test

SBN–Single-Breath Nitrogen

SBO–Small-Bowel Obstruction

SBP–Scleral Buckling Procedure; Spontaneous Bacterial Peritonitis; Systemic Blood Pressure

SBS–Social-Breakdown Syndrome; Small-Bowel Syndrome

SBSRT–Spreen-Benton Sentence Repetition Test

SC–Closure of Semilunar Valves; Sacrococcygeal; Sickle Cell; Skin Conductance; Slow Component; Snellen's Chart; Splenic Collateral; Sternoclavicular; Stimulus, Conditioned; Subclavian; Sugar Coated

SCA–Selective Coronary Angiogram; Sickle-Cell Anemia; Subcutaneous Abdominal Block

SCAB–Streptozocin, Lomustine, Adriamycin and Bleomycin

SCBC–Small-Cell Bronchogenic Carcinoma

SCC–Short-Course Chemotherapy; Sickle-Cell Crisis; Small-Cell Cancer; Squamous-Cell Carcinoma

SCD–Sequential Compression Device; Sickle-Cell Disease; Spinal Cord Disease; Subacute Combined Degeneration; Sudden Cardiac Death

ScDA–Scapuladextra Anterior Position

ScDP–Scapuladextra Posterior Position

SCE–Secretory Carcinoma of the Endometrium

SCFE–Slipped Capital Femoral Epiphysis

SCI–Spinal Cord Injury; Structured Clinical Interview

SCID–Severe Combined Immune Deficiency

SCIPP–Sacrococcygeal to Inferior Pubic Point

SCIV–Subclavian Intravenous Line

SCJ–Sclerocorneal Junction; Squamocolumnar Junction

SCL–Scleroderma

SCLE–Subacute Cutaneous Lupus Erythematosus

SCM–Spondylitic Caudal Myelopathy; Sternocleidomastoid Muscle

SCR–Skin Conductance Response; Spondylitic Caudal Radioculopathy

SCRAP–Simple Complex Reaction-Time Apparatus

SCT–Sentence Completion Test; Sickle-Cell Trait; Staphylococcal Clumping Test; Sugar-Coated Tablet

SCUT–Schizophrenia, Chronic Undifferentiated Type

SCV–Subcutaneous Vaginal Block

SCWT–Stroop Color-Word Test

SD–Senile Dementia; Septal Defect; Serum Defect; Shoulder Disarticulation; Skin Destruction; Skin Dose; Spontaneous Delivery; Sterile Dressing; Stone Disintegration; Sudden Death; Systolic Discharge

S&D–Stomach and Duodenum

SDA–Sacrodextra Anterior Position; Specific Dynamic Action of Foods; Steroid Dependent Asthmatic

SDAT–Senile Dementia, Alzheimer Type

SDH–Spinal Dorsal Horn; Subdural Hematoma

SDHD–Sudden Death Heart Disease

SDL–Serum Digoxin Level

SDM–Sensory Detection Method

SDP–Sacrodextra Position

SDS–Sensory Deprivation Syndrome; Sudden Death Syndrome

SDT–Sacrodextra Transversa; Spache Diagnostic Test; Speech Detection Threshold

SDU–Short Double Upright Brace

SE–Saline Enema; Stage of Exhaustion; Starr-Edwards Prosthesis

Se–Selenium (Chemical Symbol)

SEA–Sheep Erythrocyte Agglutination; Spontaneous Electrical Activity

SEBA–Staphylococcal Enterotoxin B Antiserum

SED–Skin Erythema Dose; Spondyloepiphyseal Dysplasia

SEEP–Small End-Expiratory Pressure

SEF–Somatically Evoked Field

SEG–Sonoencephalogram

SEI–Superficial Epithelial Infiltrates

SEM–Soft Ejection Murmur; Somatosensory Evoked Potential; Systolic Ejection Murmur

SEMI–Subendocardial Myocardial Infarction

SEMLSB–Systolic Ejection Murmur, Left Sternal Border

SEP–Sensory Evoked Potential; Sperm Entry Point; Systolic Ejection Period

SER–Somatosensory Evoked Resonse; Systolic Ejection Rate

SES–Spatial Emotional Stimuli

SET–Systolic Ejection Time

SF–Salt-Free; Scarlet Fever; Semi-Fowler's Position; Seminal Fluid; Serum Fibrinogen; Spinal Fluid; Sterile Female; Stress Formula; Synovial Fluid

SFA–Saturated Fatty Acids; Superficial Femoral Artery

SFC–Soluble Fibrin-Fibrinogen Complex; Spinal Fluid Count

SFD–Short Food Drape; Skin-Film Distance

SFEMG–Single-Fiber Electromyography

SFFF–Sedimentation Field Flow Fractionization

SFO–Subfornical Organ

SFP–Simultaneous Foveal Perception; Spinal Fluid Pressure

SFS–Skin and Fascial Stapler

SG–Sachs-Georgi Test; Skin Graft; Specific Gravity; Swan-Ganz Catheter

SGA–Small for Gestational Age

SGAW–Specific Airway Conductance

SGC–Spermicide-Germicide Compound

SGD–Straight Gravity Drainage

SGE–Significant Glandular Enlargement

SGFR–Single-Nephron Glomerular Filtration Rate

SGOT–Serum Glutamic Oxalo-Acetic Transaminase

SGPT–Serum Glutamic Pyruvic Transaminase

SGR–Sachs-Georgi Reaction

SH–Serum Hepatitis; Sexual Harassment; Somatotropic Hormone; Surgical History; Spontaneously Hypertensive

S&H–Speech and Hearing

SHB–Subacute Hepatitis with Bridging

SHDI–Supraorbital Hypophysial

SHEENT–Skin, Hair, Eyes, Ears, Nose and Throat

SHG–Sauerbruch, Herrmannsdorfer, Gerson Diet; Synthetic Human Gastrin

SHHP–Semihorizontal Heart Position

SHN–Spontaneous Hemorrhagic Necrosis; Subacute Hepatic Necrosis

SHS–Sayre Head Sling; Shipley-Hartford Scale

SHT–Simple Hypocalcemic Tetany; Subcutaneous Histamine Test

SI–Sacroiliac; Saline Injection; Serum Iron; Sex Inventory; Soluble Insulin; Stress Incontinence; Stroke Index; Suicidal Ideation

S&I–Suction and Irrigation

SIA–Stress-Induced Anesthesia

SIADH–Syndrome of Inappropriate Antidiuretic Hormone

SIB–Self-Injurious Behavior

SICD–Sequenced Inventory of Communicative Development

SICSVA–Sequential Impaction Cascade Sieve Volumetric Air

SICT–Selective Intracoronary Thrombolysis

SICU–Surgical Intensive Care Unit

SID–Sudden Infant Death

SIDS–Sudden Infant Death Syndrome

SIJ–Sacroiliac Joint

SILS–Shipley Institute of Living Scale

SIMV–Synchronized Intermittent Mandatory Ventilation

SIS–Sterile Injectable Suspension

SISI–Short Increment Sensitivity Index

SIT–Slossen Intelligence Test; Sperm Immobilization Test

SJ–Stevens-Johnson Test

SK–Senile Keratosis; Solar Keratosis; Streptokinase; Striae Keratopathy

SKA–Supracondylar Knee-Ankle

SKAT–Sex Knowledge and Aptitude

SL–Sensation Level; Sinding Larsen; Sjogren-Larsson; Slit Lamp; Small Lymphocyte; Sound Level; Stein-Leventhal Syndrome; Strumpell-Lorrain Disease; Sublingual

SLA–Sacrolaeva Anterior Position

SLAP–Serum Leucine Aminopeptidase

SLB–Short-Leg Brace

SLC–Short-Leg Cast

SLDS–Single-Level Dynamic Scanner

SLE–Saint Louis Encephalitis; Slit Lamp Examination; Systemic Lupus Erythematosus

SLGXT–Symptom-Limited Graded Exercise Test

SLI–Splenic Localization Index

SLK–Superior Limbic Keratoconjunctivitis

SLN–Superior Laryngeal Nerve

SLP–Sacrolaeva Posterior Position

SLR–Straight-Leg Raising

SLRT–Straight-Leg-Raising Tenderness

SLS–Short-Leg Splint

SLT–Sacrolaeva Transversa Position

SM–Sadomasochism; Self-Monitoring; Semimembranous; Simple Mastectomy; Smooth Muscle; Stapedius Muscle; Submandibular; Submucosal; Suction Method; Superior Mesenteric; Supramamillary; Synaptic Membrane; Synovial Membrane; Systolic Mean; Systolic Murmur

SMA–Spinal Muscular Atrophy; Superior Mesenteric Artery

SMAO–Superior Mesenteric Artery Occlusion

SMAS–Superficial Musculoaponeurotic System

SMC–Special Mouth Care; Succinylmonocholine

SMD–Senile Macular Degeneration; Submanubrial Dullness

SMF–Streptozocin, Mitomycin-C; and 5-Fluorouracil

SMI–Style of Mind Inventory; Sustained Maximal Inspiration

SMON–Subacute Myelo-Optical Neuropathy

SMR–Sensorimotor Rhythm; Skeletal Muscle Relaxant; Submucosal Resection

SMRR–Submucous Resection and Rhinoplasty

SMV–Submento-Vertex View

SMVT–Sustained Monomorphic Ventricular Tachycardia

SMZ-TMP–Sulfamethoxazole and Trimethoprim

SN–Sensory Neuron; Sinus Node; Sternal Notch; Streptonigran; Suprasternal Notch

SNAP–Sensory Nerve Action Potential

SNCV–Sensory Nerve Conduction Velocity

SND–Sinus Node Dysfunction

SNE–Spatial Nonemotional Stimuli; Subacute Necrotizing Encephalomyelopathy

SNHL–Sensorineural Hearing Loss

SNP–Sodium Nitroprusside

SNR–Signal-to-Noise Ratio

SNS–Sympathetic Nervous System

SNT–Sinuses, Nose and Throat

SNV–Spleen Necrosis Virus

SO–Salpingo-Oophorectomy; Spheno-Occipital; Superior Oblique; Supraoptic

SOA–Supraorbital Artery; Swelling of Ankle

SOAP–Subjective Data, Objective Data, Assessment and Plan

SOB–Shortness of Breath; Suboccipitobregmatic Sutures

SOC–Sequential-Type Oral Contraceptive

SOM–Secretory Otitis Media

SOMI–Skull Occipital Mandibular Immobilization; Sterno-Occipital Mandibular Immobilization

SONK–Spontaneous Osteonecrosis of the Knee

SONP–Solid Organs Not Palpable

SORT–Slosson Oral Reading Test

SOS–Supplemental Oxygen System

SP–Sacrum Posterior Position; Shunt Procedure; Skin Potential; Speech Pathology; Steady Potential; Suicide Precautions; Suprapubic; Symphysis Pubis; Systolic Pressure

SPA–Salt-Poor Albumin; Stimulation-Produced Analgesia; Suprapubic Aspiration

SPAD–Subcutaneous Peritoneal Access Device

SPBT–Suprapubic Bladder Tap

SPC–Salicyamide, Phenacetin and Caffeine; Standard Platelet Count

SPFT–Sixteen Personality Factors Test

SPG–Sphenopalatine Ganglion

SPH–Secondary Pulmonary Hemosiderosis; Severely and Profoundly Handicapped

SPI–Stuttering Prediction Instruction

SPK–Superficial Punctate Keratitis

SPL–Skin Potential Level; Sound Pressure Level; Spontaneous Lesion

SPMA–Spinal Progressive Muscle Atrophy

SPMB–Strong Partial Maternal Behavior

SPMI–Status Post Myocardial Infarction

SPN–Sympathetic Preganglionic Neuron

SPO–Status Postoperative

SPP–Sexuality Preference Profile; Suprapubic Prostatectomy

SPR–Serial Probe Recognition

SPROM–Spontaneous Premature Rupture of Membranes

SPTI–Systolic Pressure Time Index

SPTURP–Status Post Transurethral Resection of the Prostate

SPVR–Systemic Peripheral Vascular Resistance

SQ–Social Quotient; Subcutaneous

SR–Sedimentation Rate; Seizure Resistant; Sensitivity Response; Sinus Rhythm; Skin Resistance; Stage of Resistance; Stomach Rumble; Stretch Reflex; Superficial Reflex; Superior Rectus; Surgical Removal; Sustained Release; Systemic Resistance

SRC–Sedimented Red Cell; Social Rehabilitation Center

SRF–Skin Respiratory Factor; Somatotropin-Releasing Factor; Split Renal Function; Subretinal Fluid

SRH–Single Radical Hemolysis; Spontaneously Resolving Hyperthyroidism

SRM–Superior Rectus Muscle

SRN–Subretinal Neovascularization

SRS–Silver-Russell Syndrome; Slow-Reacting Substance

SRT–Sedimentation Rate Test; Sinus Node Recovery Time; Social Relations Test; Speech Reception Test; Sustained-Release Theophylline

SS–Saline Solution; Schizophrenia Spectrum; Seizure Sensitive; Serum Sickness; Side-to-Side; Skull Series; Somatostatin; Stable Sarcoidosis; Staccato Syndrome; Standard Score; Strachan-Scott Syndrome; Subaortic Stenosis; Sunsegmental; Substernal; Systemic Sclerosis

S&S–Signs and Symptoms; Support and Stimulation

SSA–Skin-Sensitizing Antibody

SSCA–Single Shoulder Contrast Arthrography

SSCT–Sacks Sentence Completion Test

SSD–Source-Skin Distance

SSE–Saline Solution Enema; Skin Self-Examination; Systemic Side Effects

SSEP–Somatosensory Evoked Potential

SSFP–Steady-State Free Precession

SSI–Stuttering Severity Index; Subshock Insulin; Synthetic Sentence Identification; System Sign Inventory

SSIDS–Sibling of Sudden Infant Death Syndrome

SSKI–Saturated Solution of Potassium Iodide

SSM–Subsynaptic Membrane; Superficial Spreading Melanoma

SSP–Subacute Sclerosing Panencephalitis; Supersentivity Perception

SSPE–Subacute Sclerosing Panencephalitis

SSPL–Saturation Sound Pressure Level

SSS–Sick Sinus Syndrome; Sterile Saline Soak; Strong Soap Solution

SSSS–Staphylococcal Scalded Skin Syndrome

SSV–Simian Sarcoma Virus

SSW–Staggered Spondiac Word Test

ST–Sedimentation Time; Sinus Tachycardia; Skin Test; Speech Therapist; Sphincter Tone; Split Thickness; Sternothyroid; Stress Testing; Subtalar; Superior Turbinate

STA–Serum Thrombotic Accelerator; Superficial Temporal Artery

STAG–Split Thickness Autogenous Graft

STC–Soft Tissue Calcification

STD–Sexually Transmitted Disease; Skin Test Dose; Skin to Tumor Distance; Standard Test Dose

STET–Submaximal Treadmill Exercise Test

STG–Short-Term Goal; Split Thickness Graft

STH–Soft Tissue Hematoma

STI–Systolic Time Interval

STJ–Subtalar Joint

STL–Swelling, Tenderness and Limitation

STM–Short-Term Memory; Streptomycin

STNR–Symmetrical Tonic Neck Reflex

STORCH–Syphilis, Toxoplasmosis, Other Agents, Rubella, Cytomegalovirus and Herpes

STS–Serological Test for Syphilis; Soft-Tissue Swelling; Subtrapezial Space

STT–Scaphotrapeziotrapezoid Joint; Serial Thrombin Time; Standard Triple Therapy

STVA–Subtotal Villose Atrophy

SU–Sensation Unit; Sensory Urgency

S&U–Supine and Upright

SUA–Sedative Urinary Antibiotic; Single Umbilical Artery

SUB–Skene's, Urethral and Bartholin's

SUDS–Subjective Units of Distress

SUF–Sequential Unexplained Infant Death

SUN–Serum Urea Nitrogen

SUS–Stained Urinary Sediment

SUX–Succinylcholine

SV–Sarcoma Virus; Scalp Vein; Sigmoid Volvulus; Single Ventricle; Sinus Venous; Spoken Voice; Stroke Volume; Subclavian Vein; Supraventricular

SVAS–Supravalvular Aortic Stenosis

SVBPG–Saphenous Vein Bypass Graft

SVC–Slow Vital Capacity; Superior Vena Cava

SVCG–Spatial Vectorcardiogram

SVCO–Superior Vein Cava Obstruction

SVCS–Superior Vena Cava Syndrome

SVD–Spontaneous Vaginal Delivery; Spontaneous Vertex Delivery

SVE–Sterile Vaginal Examination

SVG–Saphenous Vein Graft

SVI–Stroke Volume Index

SVM–Synctiovascular Membrane

SVN–Small Volume Nebulizer

SVPB–Supraventricular Paroxysmal Tachycardia

SVR–Supraventricular Rhythm; Systemic Vascular Resistance

SVRI–Systemic Vascular Resistance Index

SVT–Supraventricular Tachyarrhythmia; Supraventricular Tachycardia

SW–Schwartz–Watson; Slow Wave; Sterile Water

SWD–Short-Wave Diathermy

SWE–Slow-Wave Encephalography

SWFI–Sterile Water For Injection

SWIM–Sperm-Washing Insemination Method

SWS–Slow-Wave Sleep; Sturge-Weber Syndrome

Sx–Signs; Surgery; Symptoms

SYC–Small, Yellow, Constipated

SZ–Schizophrenia; Seizure; Suction

SZN–Streptozicin

T

T–Intraocular Tension; Thoracic; Thorax; Thrill; Thymus-Derived; Tidal Gas; Torque; Toxicity

TA–Temperature, Axillary; Tendo Achilis; Tension Applanation; Test of Articulation; Thoracoabdominal; Thyroid Autoantibody; Toxim-Antitoxin; Transplantation Antigen; Tricuspid Atresia; Truncus Arteriosus; Tuberculin, Alkaline; Tumor-Associated

T & A–Tonsillectomy and Adenoidectomy

TAA–Thoracic Aortic Aneurysm; Total Ankle Arthroscopy

TAB–Theraputic Abortion; Triple Antibiotic; Typhoid, Paratyphoid A, and Paratyphoid B

TABT–Combined Typhoid, Paratyphoid A, and Paratyphoid B, and Tetanus Toxoid

TABTD–Combined Typhoid, Paratyphoid A, and Paratyphoid B, Tetanus Toxoid, and Diphtheria Toxoid

TAC–Terminal Atrial Contraction; Triamcinolone Cream

TACL–Test for Auditory Comprehension of Language

TAD–Thioguanine, Cystosine Arabinoside, and Daunomycin; Thoracic Asphyxiant Dystrophy; Transverse Abdominal Diameter

TADAC–Therapeutic Abortion, Dilation, Aspiration, Curettage

TAE–Transcatheter Arterial Embolization

TAH–Total Abdominal Hysterectomy; Total Artificial Heart; Transabdominal Hysterectomy

TALTFR–Teno(or Tendo) Achillis Lengthening and Toe Flexor Release

TANI–Total Axial (Lymph) Node Irradiation

TAO–Thromboangitis Obliterans

TAPVC–Total Anomalous Pulmonary Venous Connection

TAPVR–Total Anomalous Pulmonary Venous Return

TAR–Thrombocytopenia With Absent Radius; Total Ankle Replacement

TARA–Total Articular Replacement Arthroplasty

TAT–Thematic Apperception Test; Thromboplastin Activation Time; Till All Taken

TATST–Tetanus Antitoxin Skin Test

TB–Terminal Bronchiole; Thromboxane B; Tracheal Bronchiolar; Tracheobronchitis; Trapezoid Body; Tubercle Bacillus; Tuberculin; Tuberculosis

TBA–Testosterone-Binding Affinity; Tubercle Bacillus

TBB–Transbronchial Biopsy

TBC–Thyroxine-Binding Coagulin

TBE–Tick-Born Encephalitis; Tuberculin Bacillary Emulsion

TBG–Testosterone-Binding Globulin; Thyroglobulin

TBGP–Total Blood Granulocyte Pool

TBH–Total Body Hematocrit

TBI–Thyrobinding Index; Tooth Brushing Instruction; Total Body Irradiation; Traumatic Brain Injury

TBLB–Transbronchial Lung Brush

TBLC–Term Birth, Living Child

TBLI–Term Birth Living Infant

TBM–Tuberculous Meningitis; Tubular Basement Membrane

TBN–Bacillus Emulsion

TBP–Testosterone-Binding Protein; Tyberculous Peritonitis

TBT–Tracheobronchial Toilet

TBTNR–Toronto Biculture Test of Nonverbal Reasoning

TBV–Total Blood Volume; Transluminal Balloon Valvuloplasty

TC–Tetracycline; Thoracic Cage; Throat Culture;Thyrocalcitonin; Total Capacity; Total Colonoscopy; Transcutaneous; True Conjugate; Tuberculin, Contagious; Tubocurarine; Type and Crossmatch

T & C–Turn and Cough; Type and Cross

TCA–Terminal Carcinoma; Transluminal Coronary Angioplasty; Trichloroacetic Acid; Tricuspid Atresia; Tricyclic Antidepressant

T-CAP–Baker's Antifol, Cyclophosphamide, Adriamycin, and Cisplatin

TCB–Total Cardiopulmonary Bypass; Tumor Cell Burden

TCC–Thromboplaxtic Cell Component

TCCB–Transitional-Cell Carcinoma of Bladder

TCDB–Turn, Cough, and Deep Breath

TCES–Transcutaneous Cranial Electrial Stimulation

TCF–Total Coronary Flow

TCGF–Thymus Cell Growth Factor

TCH–Total Circulating Hemoglobin; Turn, Cough, and Hyperventilate

TCI–Transient Cerebral Ischemia

TCIE–Transient Cerebral Ischemic Episode

TCMH–Tumor-Direct Cell-Mediated Hypersensitivity

T-COPA–Vincristine, Prednisone, Cytosine Arabinoside, Cyclophosphamide, and 6-Thioguanine

TCOM–Transcutaneous Oxygen Monitor

TCP–Therapeutic Continuous Penicillin

TCR–Thalamocortical Relay

TCT–Thrombin-Clotting Time

TCV–Thoracic Cage Volume

TD–Takayasu's Disease; Tardive Dyskinesia; Tetanus and Diphtheria; Therapy Discontinued; Thoracic Duct; Threshold Dose; Thymus-Dependent; Tone Delay; Total Dose; Transverse Diameter; Traveler's Diarrhea; Treating Distance; Tuberoinfundobular Dopaminergic; Tumor Dose; Typhoid-Dysentery

TDD–Thoracic Duct Drainage

TDE–Total Digestible Energy

TDF–Thoracic Duct Fistula; Thoracic Duct Flow; Tumor Dose Fractionation

TDK–Tardive Dyskinesia

TDL–Thoracic Duct Lymph; Thymus-Dependent Lymphocyte

TDM–Theraputic Drug Monitoring

TDP–Thoracic Duct Pressure

TDT–Tentative Drainage Tomorrow; Tone Decay Test

TDTA–Templin Darley Test of Articulation

TTDWB–Touch-Down Weight-Bearing

TE–Tennis Elbow; Test Ear; Thromboembolism; Thymus Epithelial; Thyrotoxic Exophthalmos; Tooth Extracted; Tracheoesophageal Treadmill Exercise

TEA–Thromboendarterectomy; Total Elbow Arthroplasty

TEC–Total Eosinophil Count; Transient Erythroblastopenia of Childhood

TED–Tasks of Emotional Development; Threshold Erythema Dose; Thromboembolic Disease

TEE–Transesophageal Echocardiography

TEF–Tetralogy of Fallot; Tracheoesophageal Fistula; Trunk Extension-Flexion

TEG–Thromboelastogram

TEN–Total Enteral Nutrition; Toxic Epidermal Necrolysis

TENS–Transcutaneous Electrical Nerve Stimulation

TEP–Thromboendophlebectomy

TER–Total Endoplasmic Reticulum; Transcapillary Escape Rate

TES–Transmural Electrical Stimulation

TET–Tetralogy of Fallot; Treadmill Exercise Test

TEV–Talipes Equinovarus

TF–Tactile Fremitus; Tetralogy of Fallot; Tracheal Fistula; Transfer Factor; Tuberculin Filtrate

TFB–Trifascicular Block

TFEV–Timed Forced Expiratory Volume

TFL–Tensor Fascia Lata

Tfm–Testicular Feminization Syndrome

TFN–Total Fecal Nitrogen

TFT–Thyroid Function Tests; Tight Fingertip; Transfer Factor Test

TG–Tendon Graft; Thromboglobulin; Thyroglobulin; Toxic Goiter

TGA–Transient Global Amnesia; Transposition of the Great Arteries

TGAR–Total Graft Area Rejected

TGC–Time Gain Compensation

TGE–Transmissible Gastroenteritis

Tgf–Transformin Growth Factor

TGR–Tenderness, Guarding, Rigidity

TGT–Thromboplastin Generation Test

TGV–Thoracic Gas Volume; Transposition of the Great Vessels

TH–Thoracic; Thrill; Thyrohyoid; Thyroid Hormone; Total Hysterectomy

THA–Total Hip Arthroplasty; Transient Hemispheric Attack

THC–Transhepatic Cholangiogram

THF–Thymic Humoral Factor

THI–Transient Hypogammaglobinemia of Infancy

THM–Total Heme Mass

THR–Target Heart Rate; Total Hip Replacement

THSC–Totipotent Hematopoietic Stem Cell

TI–Terminal Ileum; Thalassemia Intermedia; Thoracic Index; Tissue Invasiveness; Transverse Inlet; Tricuspid Incompetence

TIA–Transient Ischemic Attack

TIBC–Total Iron-Binding Capacity

TID–Ter In Die; Titrated Initial Dose

TIE–Transient Ischemic Episode

TIF–Tumor-Inducing Factor

TIG–Tetanus Immune Globulin

TIM–Transthoracic Intracardiac Monitoring

TIMC–Tumor-Induced Cytatocity

TIS–Tetracycline-Induced Steatosis

TIUV–Total Intrauterine Volume

TIVC–Thoracic Inferior Vena Cava

TIW–Three Times a Week

TJ–Tendon Jerk; Triceps Jerk; Troell-Junet Syndrome

TJN–Twin Jet Nebulizer

TJR–Total Joint Replacement

TDA–Total Knee Arthroplasty

TKD–Tokodynamometer

TKP–Thermokeratoplasty

TKO–To Keep Open

TKR–Total Knee Replacement

TL–Temporal Lobe; Thymic Lymphoma; Thymus Leukemia; Thymus Lymphoma; Tubal Ligation

TLA–Translumbar Aortogram; Transluminal Angioplasty

TLC–Total Lung Capacity; Total Lymphocyte Count

TLD–Thoracic Lymph Duct; Tumor Lethal Dose

TLE–Temproal Lobe Epilepsy

TLI–Total Lymphoid Irradiation

TLS–Thoracolumbosacral Drain

TLV–Threshold Limit Value: Total Lung Volume

TM–Temporomandibular; Thalassemia Major; Time-Motion Technique; Transcendental Meditation; Transitional Mucosa; Transmediastinal; Transmetatarsal; Tympanic Membrane;

T&M–Trichomonas and Monilia

TMA–Thyroid Microsomal Antibody; Transmetatarsal Amputation

TMB–Transient Monocular Blindness

TMC–Transmural Colitis

TME–Total Metabolizable Energy

TMG–Maximum Tubular Reabsorption Rate for Glucose (of Kidney)

TMI–Threatened Myocardial Infarction; Transmural Infarction

TMJ–Temporomandibular Joint

T-MOP–Methotrexate, 6-Thioguanine, Vincristine, and Prednisone

TMP–Transmembrane Potential; Transmembrane Pressure

TMR–Topical Magnetic Resonance; Trainable Mentally Retarded

TMS–Thallium Myocardial Scintigraphy;Trimethoprim and Sulfamethoxazole

TMT–Tarsometatarsal Joint; Trail Making Test

TMTC–Too Many To Count

TN–Team Nursing

Tn–Intraocular Tension; Normal Intraocular Pressure

TND–Term Normal Delivery

TNF–Tumor Necrosis Factor

TNG–Nitroglycerin

TNI–Total Nodal Irradiation

TNR–Tonic Neck Reflex

TNS–Transcutaneous Nerve Stimulation

TNTC–Too Numerous To Count

TO–Target Organ; Tuberculin Ober; Tubo-Ovarian

TOA–Time Of Arrival; Tubo-Ovarian Abcess

TOAP–Thioguanine, Oncovin (Vincristine), Cytosine Arabinoside (Cytarabine) and Prednisone

TOC–Tubo-Ovarian Complex

TOE–Tracheo-Oesophageal

TOF–Tetralogy of Fallot; Tracheo-Esophageal Fistula

TOGV–Transposition of Great Vessels

TOP–Termination of Pregnancy; Transovarial Passage

TOPV–Trivalent Oral Poliovirus Vaccine

TORCH–Toxoplasmosis, Rubella, Cytomegalovirus, and Herpes Simplex(Titer)

TORP–Total Ossicular Chain Replacement Prosthesis

TOS–Thoracic Outlet Syndrome

TOWER–Testing, Orientation, Work, Evaluation, Rehabilitation

TP–Temporoparietal; Terminal Phalanx; Testosterone Propionate; Threshold Potential; Thrombocytopenic Purpura; Thymic Polypeptide; Todd's Paralysis; Transverse Process; Treponema Pallidum; Trigger Point

TPA–Total Parenteral Alimentation; Treponema Pallidum Agglutination

TPBF–Total Pulmonary Blood Flow

TPC–Thromboplastic Plasma Component; Treponema Pallidum Complement

TPCV–Total Packed Cell Volume

TPD–Tropical Pancreatic Diabetes; Tumor-Producing Dose

TPE–Therapeutic Plasma Exchange; Total Protective Environment

TPG–Transmembrane Potential Gradient; Transplacental Gradient

TPH–Thromboembolic Pulmonary Hypertension; Transplacental Hemorrhage

TPHA–Treponemal Hemagglutination

TPI–Treponema Pallidum Immobilization

TPM–Temporary Pacemaker; Total Passive Motion

TPN–Thalamic Projection Neuron; Total Parenteral Nutrition

TPPN–Total Peripheral Parenteral Nutrition

TPR–Temperature, Pulse, and Respiration; Total Peripheral Resistance; Total Pulmonary Resistance

TPRI–Total Peripheral Resistance Index

TPTHS–Total Parathyroid Hormone Secretion

TPUR–Transperineal Urethral Resection

TPVR–Total Peripheral Vascular Resistance

TR–Temperature, Rectal; Therapeutic Radiology; Time Recovery; Total Resistance; Tricuspid Regurgitation

TRAM–Transverse Rectus Abdominis Myocutaneous

TRAP–Thioguanine, Rubidomycin, Ara-C, and Prednisone

TRBF–Total Renal Blood Flow

TRC–Tanned Red Cells

TRD–Traction Retinal Detachment

TRE–True Radiation Emission

TRF–Thymus-Dependent Cell Replacing Factor

TRI–Total Response Index; Tubuloreticular Inclusion

TRP–Total Refraction Period; Total Refractory Period; Trichorhinophalangeal; Tubular Reabsorption of Phosphate

TRPS–Trichorhinophalangeal Syndrome

TRPT–Theoretical Renal Phosphorus Threshold

TS–Temperature-Sensitive; Temporal Stem; Terminal(or Greater) Sensation; Thoracic Surgery; Total Solids; Tourette Syndrome;

Transsexual; Tricuspid Stenosis; Triple Strength; Tuberous Sclerosis; Tubular (Tracheal) Sound; Turner Syndrome

TSA–Technical Surgical Assistance; Test of Syntactic Abilities; Total Shoulder Arthroplasty

TSAS–Total Severity Assessment Score

TSBB–Transtracheal Selective Bronchial Brushing

TSD–Tay-Sachs Disease

TSE–Testicular Self-Examination; Total Skin Examination

TSF–Thrombopoietic Stimulating Factor; Triceps Skin Fold

TSG–Tumor-Specific Glcoprotein

TSH–Thyroid-Stimulating Glycoprotein

TSI–Thyroid-Stimulating Immunoglobulin

TSP–Teaspoon

TSPAP–Total Serum Prostatic Acid Phosphatase

TSPP–Technetium Stannous Pyrophosphate

TSR–Testosterone Sterilized (Female)Rate; Thyroid-to-Serum Ratio; Total Shoulder Replacement

TSS–Toxic Shock Syndrome; Transverse Spinal Sclerosis; Tropical Splenomegaly Syndrome

TSSA–Tumor-Specific Cell Surgace Antigen

TSSU–Theater Sterile Supply Unit

TST–Treadmill Stress Test; Tumor Skin Test

TT–Tendon Transfer; Tetanus Toxin; Thrombin Time; Thymol Turbidity; Tibial Torsion; Tibial Tubercle; Token Test; Total Thyroxine; Transient Tachypnea; Transit Time; Transthroacic; Transtracheal; Twitch Tension

T & T–Time and Temperature; Touch and Tone; Tympanostomy with Tube Placement

TTA–Total Toe Arthroplasty; Transtracheal Aspiration

TTD–Tissue Tolerance Dose

TTI–Tension-Time Index

TTIB–Tension-Time Index per Beat

TTN–Transient Tachypnea of the Newborn

TTP-Thrombotic Thrombocytopenic Purpura; Time-To-Peak

TTS–Transdermal Theraputic System

TTT–Tolbutamide Tolerance Test

TTVP–Temporary Transvenous Pacemaker

TU–Tuberculin Unit

TUB–Tubouterine (Junction)

TUD–Total Urethral Discharge

TUG–Total Urinary Gonadotropin

TUIP–Transurethral Incision of the Prostate

TUR–Transurethral Resection (of Bladder)

TURB–Transurethral Resection of the Bladder

TURBN–Transurethral Resection of the Bladder Neck

TURBT–Transurethral Resection of Bladder Tumor

TURP–Transurethral Resection of Prostate

TURV–Transurethral Resection of Valves

TV–Talipes Varus; Tidal Volume; Transvenous; Trichomonas Vaginalis; Tricuspid Valve; Truncal Vagotomy

TVC–Timed Vital Capacity; Total Vital Capacity; Transvaginal Cone; True Vocal Cords

TVD–Transmissible Virus Dementia; Triple-Vessel Disease

TVDALV–Triple-Vessel Disease with Abnormal Left Ventricle

TVF–Tactile Vocal Fremitus

TVH–Total Vaginal Hysterectomy

TVP–Transvenous Pacemaker; Transvesical Prostatectomy; Tricuspid Valve Prolapse

TVT–Tunica Vaginalis Testis

TVU–Total Volume Urine

TVV–Transmissible Venereal Virus Gynecology, Infectious Diseases

TW–Tapwater

TWD–Total White and Differential Count

TWETC–Tapwater Enema Till Clear

TWL–Transepidermal Water Loss
TX–Thromboxane; Traction; Transplant
T & X–Type and Crossmatch
TX–Therapy; Treatment

U

U–Ultralente Insulin; Unerupted; Urologist
UA–Ultra-Audible; Unstable Angina; Urinalysis; Uterine Aspiration;
UAC–Umbilical Artery Catheter
UAD–Upper–Airway Disease
UAE–Unilateral Absence of Excretion
UAL–Umbilical Artery Line
Uao–Upper-Airway Obstruction
UAVC–Univentricular Atrioventricular Connection
UB–Ultimobranchial
UBF–Uterine Blood Flow
UBG–Ultimobranchial Glands; Urobilinogen
UBI–Ultraviolet Blood Irradiation
UBO–Unidentified Bright Object
UBP–Ureteral Back Pressure
UC–Ulcerative Colitis; Urea Clearance; Urethral Catheterization;
    Urinary Catheter; Urine Culture
U & C–Urethral and Cervical
UCD–Urine-Collection Device; Usual Childhood Diseases
UCG–Ultrasonic Cardiogram; Urinary Chorionic Gonadotropin
UCI–Urinary Catheter In
UCL–Uncomfortable Loudness; Urea Clearance
UCO–Urinary Catheter Out
UCP–Urinary Coproporphyrin
UCR–Unconditioned Response

UCTD–Unclassified Connective Tissue Disease
UD–Ulcerative Dermatitis; Ulnar Deviation; Urethral Discharge
UDC–Usual Diseases of Childhood
UDS–Ultra-Doppler Sonography
UE–Uncertain Etiology; Upper Esophagus; Upper Extremity; Urinary
   Energy
UES–Upper Esophageal Sphincter
UF–Ultrafiltrable; Umbrella Filter
UG–Urogenital
UGA–Under General Anesthesia
UGH–Uveitis, Glaucoma, and Hyphema
UGI–Upper Gastrointestinal
UGS–Urogenital Sinus
UHBI–Upper Hemibody Irradiation
UHD–Unstable Hemoglobin Disease
UHL–Universal Hypertrichosis Lanuginosa
UHR–Underlying Heart Rhythm
UI–Ureteral-Intestinal
UIF–Undegraded Insulin Factor
UIP–Usual Interstital Pneumonia; Usual Interstitial Pneumonitis
UIQ–Upper Inner Quadrant
UL–Undifferentiated Lymphoma; Upper Lobe
ULBW–Ultralow Birth Weight
ULL–Uncomfortable Loudness Level
ULQ–Uper Left Quadrant
UMN–Upper Motor Neuron
UMNb–Upper Motor Neurogenic Bladder
UMNL–Upper Motor Neuron Lesion
UN–Ulnar Nerve; Urea Nitrogen; Urinary Nitrogen
UO–Ureteral Orifice; Urinary Output
UOQ–Upper Outer Quadrant
UP–Upright Posture; Ureteropelvic

UPA–Unpressurized Aerosol

UPF–Universal Proximal Femur

UPG–Uroporphyrinogen

UPI–Uteroplacental Insuffciency; Uteroplacental Ischemia

UPJ–Ureteropelvic Junction; Uteropelvic Junction

UPP–Universal Proximal Femoral Prosthesis; Urethral Pressure Profile; Uvulopalatopharyngoplasty

UPS–Uterine Progesterone System

UPT–Urine Pregnancy Test

UQ–Upper Quadrant

UR–Unconditioned Reflex; Upper Respiratory; Utilization Review

URC–Upper Rib Cage

URD–Upper Respiratory Disease

URF–Uterine-Relaxing Factor

URI–Upper Respiratory Infection

URQ–Upper Right Quadrant

URS–Ultrasonic Renal Scanning

URT–Upper Respiratory Tract

US–Ultrasonic; Unconditioned Stimulus; Urinary Space

USo-Unilateral Salpingo-Oophorectomy

USS–Ultrasound Scanning

USVMS–Urine Sample Volume Measuring System

UT–Urinary Tract

UTBG–Unbound Testosterone-Binding Globulin

UTF–Usual Throat Flora

UTI–Urinary Tract Infections

UTLD–Utah Test of Language Development

UTO–Upper Tibial Osteotomy

UU–Urine Urobilinogen

UUN–Urine Urea Nitrogen

UV–Umbilical Vein; Ureterovesical; Urinary Volume

UVC–Umbilical Vein Catheter

UVI–Ultraviolet Irradiation
UVJ–Ureterovesical Junction
UVP–Ultraviolet Photometry

V

V–Gas Volume; Tidal Volume-Mechanical; Vaccinated; Vagina; Velocity; Ventilation; Vertex; Visual Acuity; Volume; Vomiting

VA–Vacuum Aspiration; Valproic Acid; Venoarterial; Vertebral Artery Visual Acuity

VAB–Vinblastine, Actinomycin D, and Bleomycin

VAC–Ventriculoarterial Connections; Vincristine, Actinomycin D(Dactinomycin) and Cyclophosphamide

VACAR–Vincristine, Adriamycin, Cyclophosphamide, and Actinomycin D

VACTERL–Vertebral, Anal, Cardiac, Tracheoesophageal, Renal, and Limb (Defects)

VAD–Vascular Access Device; Ventricular Assist Device

VADA–Vincristine, Adriamycin, Cyclophosphamide, and Actinomycin D

VADRC–Vincristine, Adriamycin, and Cyclophosphamide

VAFAC–Vincristine, Adriamycin, 5-Fllluorouracil, Methotrexate, and Cyclophosphamide

VAH–Virilizing Adrenal Hyperplasia

VAHS–Virus-Associated Hemophagocytic Syndrome

VAIN–Vaginal Intraepithelial Neoplasia

VAKT–Visual, Association, Kinaesthetic, Tactile

VALE–Visual Acuity, Left Eye

VAM–VP-16(Etoposide) Adriamycin, and Methotrexate

VAMP–Vincristine, Actinomycin, Methotrexate, and Prednisone

VAP–Variant Angina Pectoris; Vincristine, Adriamycin, and Prednisone; Vincristine, Adriamycin, and Procarbazine

VARE–Visual Acuity, Right Eye

VAS–Vesicle Attachment Site; Visual Analougue Scale

VASC–Verbal-Auditory Screen for Children

VAT–Ventricular Activation Time; Vincristine, Cytosine Arabinoside, 6-Thioguanine, and Daunomycin; Visual Action Time; Visual Apperception Test

VATER–Vertebral Defects, Imperforate Anus, Tracheoesophageal Fistula, and Radial and Renal Dysplasia

VATH–Vinblastine, Adriamycin, ThioTEPA, and Halotensin

VB–Ventrobasal; Vertebral Body; Viable Birth; Vinblastine

VABC–Vaginal Birth After Cesarean

VBAP–Vincristine, 1,3-Bis(2Chlorethyl)-1-Nitrososurea, Adriamycin, and Prednisone

VBC–Vincristine, Bleomycin, and Cisplatin

VBD–Vinblastine, Bleomycin, and Cisplatin

VBG–Vertical Banded Gastroplasty

VBI–Vertebral Basilar Insufficiency

VBOS–Veronal-Buffered Oxalated Saline

VBMCP–Vincristine, 1, 3-Bis(2-Chhloroethyl_-1-Nitrososurea{BCNU or Carmustine},L-Phenylalanine Mustard, Cyclophosphamide, and Prednisone

VBP–Vinblastine, Bleomycin, and Cisplatin

VBS–Vertebral Basilar (Artery) System

VBT–Vertebral Body Tenderness

VC–Acuity of Color Vision; Color Vision; Vasoconstriction; Vena Cava; Venereal Case; Ventilatory Capacity; Ventral Column; Visual Capacity; Visual Cortex; Vocal Cord

VCA–Vancomycin, Colistin, and Anisomycin

VCAP–Vincristine, Cyclophosphamide, Adriamycin, and Prednisone
VCE–Vagina, Ectocervix, and Endocervix
VCC–Vasoconstrictor Center
VCF–Vincristine, 5-Fluorouracil, and Cyclophosphamide
VCG–Vectocardiogram
VCMP–Vincristine, Melphalan, Cyclophophamide, and Prednisone
VCP–Vincristine, Cyclophosphamide, and Prednisone
VCR–Vincristine Sulfate
Vcs–Vasoconstrictor Substance; Vocabulary Comprehension Scale
VCT–Venous Clotting Time
VCU–Videocystourethrography; Voiding Cysturethrogram
VCUG–Vesicoureterogram; Voiding Cystourethrogram
VD–Vascular Disease; Vasodilation; Venereal Disease; Ventricular Dilator; Viral Diarrhea
Vd–Volume Dead Air Space
VDA–Venous Digital Angiogram; Visual Discriminatory Acuity
VDAC–Vaginal Delivery After Cesarean Section
VDBR–Volume of Distribution of Bilirubin
VDC–Vasodilator Center
VDEM–Vasodepressor Material
VDF–Ventricular Diastolic Fragmentation
VDG–Venereal Disease-Gonorrhea
VDH–Valvular Disease of the Heart
VDL–Vasodepressor Lipid; Visual Detection Level
VDP–Vincristine, Daunomycin, and Prednisone
VDR–Venous Diameter Ratio
VDRL–Venereal Disease Research Laboratroy
VDRR–Vitamin D-Resistant Rickets
VDRS–Verdun Depression Rating Scale
VDS–Vasodilator Substance; Venereal Disease-Syphilis; Vindesine

VDV–Ventricular End-Diastolic Volume

VE–Vaginal Examination; Venous Emptying; Ventricular Extrasystole; Vesicular Exanthema; Viral Encephalitis; Visual Efficiency; Volume Ejection

VEA–Ventricular Ectopic Activity

VEB–Ventricular Ectopic Beat

VECG–Vector Electrocardiogram

VECP–Visually Evoked Cortical Potentials

VED–Ventricular Ectopic Depolarization; Vitral Exhaustion and Depression

VEE–Vagina, Ectocervix, and Endocervix

VEF–Ventricular Ejection Fraction

VEM–Vasoexcitor Material

VEMP–Vincristine, Cyclophosphamide(Endoxan), 6-Mercaptopurine, and Prednisone

VEP–Ventricular Escape Rhythm; Visual Evoked Potential

VER–Visual Evoked Response

VESV–Vesicular Exanthema of Swine Virus

VET–Vestigial Testis

VF–Ventricular Fibrilllation; Ventricular Fluid; Vision Field; Visual Field; Vocal Fremitus

VFAM–Vincristine, 5-Fluorouracil, Adriamycin, and Mitomycin C;

VFIT–Visual Field Intact

VFL–Ventricular Filling Pressure; Ventricular Flutter

VFP–Ventricular Fluid Pressure; Vitreous Fluorophotometry

VFT–Ventricular Fibrillation Threshold; Verbal Fluency Test

VG–Vein Graft; Ventricular Gallop; Ventrogluteal

VH–Vaginal Hysterectomy; Venous Hematocrit; Ventricular Hypertrophy; Viral Hepatitis; Visually Handicapped; Vitreous Hemorrhage

VHD–Valvular Heart Disease; Ventricular Heart Disease; Viral Hematodepressive Disease

VHDL–Very High-Density Lipoprotein

VHF–Visual Half-Field

VHP–Viral Hepatitis Panel

VI–Vaginal Irrigation; Variable Interval; Vastus Intermedius; Virgo Intacta; Viscosity Index; Visual Impariment

VIBS–Vocabulary, Information, Block Design, Similarities

VIC–Vasoinhibitory Center

VID–Vagainal Intraepithelial Dysplasia; Videodensitometry

VIF–Virus-Induced Interferon

VIN–Vaginal Intraepithelial Neoplasia

VIP–Vasoactive Intestinal Polypeptide; Venous Impedance Plethysmography; Vital Initial of Pregnancy; Voluntarily Interrupted Pregnancy

VIS–Vaginal Irrigation Smear

VISC–Vitreous Infusion Suction Cutter

VIT–Venom Immunotherapy

VKC–Vernal Deratoconjunctivitis

VKH–Vogt-Koyannagi-Harada Syndrome

VL–Ventralis Lateralis; Vision, Left

VLB–Vincaleucoblastine

VLBR–Very Low Birth Rate

VLDL–Very-Low-Density Lipoprotein

VLDS–Verbal Language Development Scale

VLH–Ventrolateral Nucleus of the Hypothalamus

VLM–Visceral Larval Migrans

VLP–Vincristine, L-Asparaginase, and Prednisone

VM–Ventricular Muscle; Vestibular Membrane; Viral Myocarditis

VMC–Vasomotor Center; VP-16(Etoposide), Methotrexate, and Citrovorum Factor

VMCG–Vector Magnetocardiogram

VMCP–Vincristine, Melphalan, Cyclophosphamide, and Prednisone

VMH–Ventromedial Hypothalamic

VMN–Ventromedial Nucleus

VMO–Vastus Medialis Oblique

VMR–Vasomotor Rhinitis

VMV–Vincristine, Methotrexate, and VP-16

VN–Vomeronasal

VNE–Verbal Nonemotional Stimuli

VNO–Vomernasal Organ

VNS–Villonodular Synovitis

VOCA–VP-16(Etoposide), Vincristine, Cyclophosphamide, and Adriamycin

VOCAB–Vincristine, VP-16(Etoposide), Cyclophosphamide, Adriamycin, and Cisplatin

VOD–Venous Occlusive Disease; Venocclusive Disease; Visio Oculus Dextra

VOM–Vomited

VOR–Vestibulo-Ocular Reflex

VOS–Visio Oculus Sinister

VOU–Visio Oculus Uterque

VP–Vapor Pressure; Variegate Porphyria; Vasopressin; Venipuncture; Venous Pressure; Ventricular-Peritoneal; Ventricular Premature; Vincristine(Oncovin) and Prednisone

V & P–Vagotomy and Pyloroplasty; Ventilation and Perfusion

VPB–Ventricular Premature Beat

VPC–Ventrucular Premature Contraction; Volume-Packed Cells

VPCMF–Vincristine, Prednisone, Cyclophosphamide, Methotrexate, and 5–Fluorouracil

VPD–Ventricular Premature Depolarization

VPI–Velopharyngeal Insufficiency

VPL–Ventral Posterolateral

VPP–Viral Porcine Pneumonia

VPS–Valvular Pulmonic Stenosis; Ventriculoperitoneal Shunt

VR–Valve Replacement; Vascular Resistance; Venous Reflux; Venous Return; Ventilation Rate; Ventral Root; Ventricular Rhythm; Verbal Reprimand; Vocal Resonance; Vocational Rehabilitation

VRI–Viral Respiratory Infection

VRV–Ventricular Residual Volume

VS–Vaccination Scar; Vagal Stimulation; Venisection; Ventricular Septum; Verbal Scale; Vesicular Sound; Vesicular Stomatitis; Villonodular Synovitis; Vital Sign; Voluntary Sterilization

VSD–Ventricular Septal Defect; Virtual Safe Dose

VSFP–Venous Stop-Flow Pressure

VSM–Vascular Smooth Muscle

VSPFT–Vitalor Screening Pulmonary Function Test

VSR–Venous Stasis Retinopathy

VSS–Vital Signs Stable

VSULA–Vaccination Scar, Upper Left Arm

VSV–Vesicular Stomatitis Virus

VSW–Ventricular Stroke Work

VT–Tidal Volume; Venous Thrombosis; Ventricular Tachycardia

V & T–Volume and Tension

VTE–Venous Thromboembolism; Vicarious Trial and Error

VTG–Volume Throacic Gas

VTX–Vertex

VU–Varicose Ulcer

VUR–Vesicoureteric Reflex
VV–Varicose Veins; Venovenous; Vesicovaginal; Vulva and Vagina
VVFR–Vesicovaginal Fistula Repair
VVOR–Visual-Vestibulo-Ocular Reflex
VW–Vessel Wall
VWD–Von Willebrand's Disease
VWM–Ventricular Wall Motion
VZ–Varicella Zoster
V-Z–Varicella-Zoster
VZIG–Varicella Zoster Immune Globulin
VZV–Varicella Zoster Virus

W

W–Mechanical Work of Breathing; Water; Veight; Word Fluency; Work
WA–When Awake
WAB–Western Aphasia Battery
WACH–Wedge Adjustable Cushioned Heel
WAIS–Wechsler Adult Intelligence Scale
WAK–Wearable Artificial Kidney
WAP–Wandering Atrial Pacemaker
WAPT–Weidels Auditory Processing Test
WAS–Wiskott-Aldrich Syndrome
WB–Wechsler-Bellevue; Weight Bearing; Whole Blood
WBAPTT–Whole Blood Activated Partial Thromboplastin Time
WBAT–Weight-Bearing as Tolerated
WBC–Weight-Bearing with Crutches; Whole Blood Cell Count; White Blood Cells
WBCT–Whole Blood Clotting Time
WBH–Whole Blood Hematocrit; Whole Body Hyperthermia

WB-I Wecshsler–Bellevue I Test

WBN–Wellborn Nursery; Wide Band Noise

WBR–Whole Body Radiation

WBS–Whole Body Scan; Whole Body Shower; Withdrawal Body Shakes

WC–White Cell; Whooping Cough; Work Capacity

WCST–Wisconsin Card Sorting Test

WD–Wet Dressing; Wrist Disarticualtion

WDHA–Watery Diarrhea, Hypokalemia, and Achlorhydria

WDLL–Well-Differentiated Lymphatic Lymphoma

WF–Weil-Felix; Wet Film

WFE–Williams Flexion Exercises

WFI–Water For Injection

WFL–Within Functional Limits

WG–Wegener's Granulomatosis

WHB–Weight-Bearing

WHVP–Wedged Hepatic Venous Pressure

WISC–Wechsler Intelligence Scale for Children

WIST–Whitaker Index of Schizophrenic Thinking

WJPB–Woodcock-Johnson Psychoeducational Battery

WKD–Wilson–Kimmelstiel Disease

WKS–Wernicke-Korsakoff Syndrome

WL–Work Load

WLS–Wet Lung Syndrome

WMA–Wall Motion Abnormality

WMR–Work Metabolic Rate

WMS–Wechsler Memory Scale

WMX–Whirlpool, Message, and Exercise

WNE–West Nile Encephalitis

WOB–Work of Breathing
WP–Wetable Powder
WPFM–Wright Peak Flow Meter
Wpk–Ward's Mechanical Tissue Pack
WPPSI–Wechsler Preschool and Primary Scale of Intelligence
WPRS–Wittenborn Psychiatric Rating Scale
WPSI–Wahler Physical Symptoms Inventory
WPT–Warbled Pure Tone
WPW–Wolff-Parkinson-White
WR–Wasserman Reaction; Wiping Reaction; Wiping Reflex
WRAT–Wide Range Achievement Test
WRE–Whole Ragweed Extract
WRMT–Woodcock Reading Mastery Test
WRVP–Water Soluable; Water Swallow Williams Syndrome
WSOJ–Whole Blood Serum of a Patient with Obstructive Jaundice
WTAD–Wepman Test of Auditory Discrimination
WV–Whispered Voice
WV-MBC–Walking Ventilation to Maximum Breathing Capacity
WWAC–Walk With Aid of Cane
WY / NRT–Weidels Yes / No Reliability Test
Wza–Wide Zone Alpha

X

X–Cross; Exorphia; Removal Of; Transverse
XCCE–Extracapsular Cataract Extraction
XDP–Xeroderma Pigmentosum
XEF–Excess Ejection Fraction
XGP–Xanthogranulomatous Pyelonephritis
XP–Xeroderma Pigmentosum
XR–Roentgen Ray

XS–Cross-Section; Xiphisternum

Y

YAG–Yttrium Aluminum Garnet
YET–Youth Effectiveness Training
YF–Yellow Fever
YJV–Yellow Jacket Venom
YLC–Youngest Living Child
YO–Years Old
YORA–Younger-Onset Rheumatoid Arthritis
YPLL Years Of Potential Life Lost
YSC–Yolk Sac Carcinoma

Z

ZDS–Zung Depression Scale
ZE–Zollinger-Ellison Syndrome
ZEEP–Zero End-Expiratory Pressure
ZG–Zona Glomerulosa
ZMC–Zygomatic; Zygomaticomaxillary
ZPLS–Zimmerman Preschool Language Scale
ZR–Zona Reticularis

CONSTANTS

CONSTANTS

FACTORS TO MULTIPLY	PREFIX	SYMBOL
10^6	Mega	M
10^3	Kilo	K
10^1	Deka	da
10^{-1}	Deci	d
10^{-2}	Centi	c
10^{-3}	Milli	m
10^{-6}	Micro	μ
10^{-9}	Nano	η

SCIENTIFIC NOTATION

$$1 \times 10^{-1} = 0.1$$
$$1 \times 10^{-2} = 0.01$$
$$1 \times 10^{-3} = 0.001$$
$$1 \times 10^{-6} = 0.000001$$
$$1 \times 10^{-9} = 0.000000001$$

CONVERSIONS

Angstrom $\Rightarrow$ Meter	$\times 1.0 \times 10^{+10}$
Calorie $\Rightarrow$ Joule	$\times 4.19$
Celsius $\Rightarrow$ Farenheit	$t_F = (9/5)(t_C + 32)$
Celsius $\Rightarrow$ Kelvin	$t_K = t_C + 273.15$
Centimeter of H_2O $\Rightarrow$ Millimeter of Mercury (Hg)	$\times 0.735$
Centimeter $\Rightarrow$ Inches	$\times 0.3937$
Cup $\Rightarrow$ Meter^3	$\times 2.365882 \times 10^{-4}$
Day $\Rightarrow$ Second	$\times 86400 \ (8.64 \times 10^4)$

Dram (avoirdupois) ⇒ Kilogram	x 1.7718 x 10^{-3}
Dram (troy or apothecary) ⇒ Kilogram	x 3.8879 x 10^{-3}
Dram (U.S.Fluid) ⇒ Meter^3	x 3.69669 x 10^{-6}
Electron Volt ⇒ Joule	x 1.6021917 x 10^{-19}
Farenheit ⇒ Kelvin	$t_k = (5/9) (t_F + 459.67)$
Farenheit ⇒ Celius	$t_c = (5/9) (t_F - 32)$
Fluid Ounce ⇒ Meter^3	x 2.957352 x 10^{-5}
Foot ⇒ Meter	x 3.048 x 10^{-1}
Foot^3 ⇒ Meter^3	x 2.831684 x 10^{-2}
Gallon ⇒ Meter^3 (U.K.)	x 4.546087cx 10^{-3}
Gallon ⇒ Meter^3 (U.S.)	x 3.785411784 x 10^{-3}
Grain ⇒ Kilogram	x 6.479891 x 10^{-5}
Gram ⇒ Kilogram	x 1.0 x 10^{-3}
Inch ⇒ Centimeter	x 2.54
Inch ⇒ Meter	x 2.54 x 10^{-2}
Inch^3 ⇒ Meter^3	x 1.638706 x 10^{-5}
Joule ⇒ Calorie	+ 4.19
Kilogram ⇒ Pound	x 2.204
Liter ⇒ Meter^3	x 1.0 x 10^{-3}
Micron ⇒ Meter	x 1.0 x 10^{-6}
Mile ⇒ Meter	x 1.609 x 10^{3}
Millimeter of Hg ⇒ Centimeter of H$_2$O	x 1.36
Millimeter of Hg ⇒ PSI	x 0.0193
Ounce (Fluid) ⇒ Meter^3	x 2.9573529 x 10^{-5}

CONVERSIONS CONTINUED

Ounce (Avoirdupois) ⇒ Kilogram	x 2.834952 x 10^{-2}
Poise ⇒ Newton second/Meter^2	x 3.110347 x 10^{-2}
Pound ⇒ Kilogram	x 0.4536
Pounds per Square Inch ⇒ Millimeter Hg	x 51.71
Scruple (Apothecary) ⇒ Kilogram	x 1.0 x 10^{-1}
Tablespoon ⇒ Meter^3	x 1.478676 x 10^{-5}
Teaspoon ⇒ Meter^3	x 4.928921 x 10^{-6}
Yard^3 ⇒ Meter^3	x 0.7645548579

AVOIRDUPOIS SYSTEM

Kilogram =	1000 Grams
Kilogram =	2.205 Pounds
Kilogram =	564 Drams
Kilogram =	35.3 Drams
Kilogram =	15,432 Grains
Ounce =	16 Drams
Ounce =	28.35 Grams
Ounce =	437.5 Grains
Pound =	7,000 Grains
Pound =	453.6 Grains
Pound =	256 Drams
Pound =	16 Ounces
Dram =	11/32 Grains

PHARMACOLOGICAL WEIGHTS

GRAINS	GRAMS
30	2.0
15	1.0
10	0.6
7 ½	0.5
5	0.3
4	0.25
3	0.2
2 ½	0.15
2	0.12
1 ½	0.1
1	0.06
¾	0.05
½	0.03
3/8	0.025
1/3	0.02
¼	0.015
1/6	0.010
1/8	0.008
1/10	0.006
1/15	0.004
1/20	0.003
1/30	0.002
1/40	0.0015
1/60	0.001

WEIGHT CONVERSIONS

POUNDS	KILOGRAMS
1	0.45
2	0.9
3	1.35
4	1.80
5	2.25
6	2.70
7	3.15
8	3.60
9	4.05
10	4.50
20	9.0
30	13.5
40	18.0
50	22.5
60	27.0
70	31.5
80	36.0
90	40.5
100	45.0
200	90.0

LIQUID MEASUREMENTS

1 Fluid Ounce=	30 Cubic Centimeters or Millimeters
1/2 Fluid Ounce =	15cc.
2 1/2 Fl.Dr.=	10cc.
2 Fl.Dr.=	8cc.
1 1/4 Fl.Dr.=	5cc.
1 Fl.Dr.=	4cc.
45 Minims =	3cc.
30 Min.=	2cc.
15 Min.=	1cc.
12 Min.=	0.75cc.
10 Min.=	0.6cc.
8 Min.=	0.5cc.
5 Min.=	0.3cc.
3 Min.=	0.2cc.
1 1/2 Min.=	0.1cc.
1 Min.=	0.06cc.
3/4 Min.=	0.05cc.
1/2 Min.=	0.03cc.

Household Measures

1 Fluid Ounce =	30 ml or cc.
1 ml or cc. =	15 Minims
1 Fluid Dram =	4 ml or cc.
20 Grains =	1 Scruple
3 Scruples =	1 Dram
16 Fluid Ounces =	1 Pint
2 Pints =	1 Quart
4 Quarts =	1 Gallon

Temperature Conversion

Centigrade	Farenheit
0^0	32^0
20^0	68^0
22^0	71.6^0
24^0	75.2^0
26^0	78.8^0
28^0	82.4^0
30^0	86^0
32^0	89.6^0
34^0	93.2^0
36^0	96.8^0
36.2^0	97.2^0
36.4^0	97.5^0
36.6^0	97.9^0
36.8^0	98.2^0
37.0^0	98.6^0
37.2^0	99^0
37.4^0	99.3^0
37.6^0	99.7^0
37.8^0	100^0
38^0	100.4^0
38.2^0	100.8^0
38.4^0	101.1^0
38.6^0	101.5^0
38.8^0	101.8^0

39.0^{0}	102.2^{0}
39.2^{0}	102.6^{0}
39.4^{0}	102.9^{0}
39.6^{0}	103.3^{0}
39.8^{0}	103.6^{0}
40.0^{0}	104.^{0}

LABORATORY VALUES

LABORATORY VALUES

The values that folow are averages. Since each laboratory varies as to technique and technologist performing the test, there are specific value ranges particluar to each institution. If a value falls near one end of the spectrum, the particular range for that institution should be checked before instituting a therapy or making a medical decision.

Level	Theraputic or Nom als
Acetom inophen	Pediatric or Adult Levels = 5-20 ug /m l or 31-124 um ol/L (S Iunits) Toxic Levels = 50 ug /m l or 200 ug /m l (hepatic Toxicity) or 305 um ol/L (S Iunits)
Acetone (acetoacetate)	Adult = 0.3-2.0 m g /dl or 51.6-344 um ol/L (S Iunits) Pediatric = 0.4-2.2 m g /dl
Acid Phosphatase	Adult = 0.5-2 U /dl (Bodansky) 0.1-5 U /dl (King -A m strong) 0.1-2 U /dl (Gutm an) 0.1-0.8 U /dl (Bessey -Low ry) 0.13-0.63 U /L (S Iunits) Prostatic = 2.5-12 IU/L New born = 10.3-16.3 U /m l (King-A m strong) Pediatric = 0.5-11 U /m l (King-A m strong) 6.4-15.2 U/L (S Iunits)
Alanine Am inotransferase (ALT)	Adult = 5-40 U /m l (Frankel) 16-60 U /m l at 30C . (Karm en) 5-25 m U /m l (W roblew ski) 4-36 U /L at 37C .(S Iunits) New born = 4 tim es the adult level Pediatric = Sam e as the adult level
Album in	3-5.5 g /dl
Alcohol Level	Adult = 0.05% or 50 m g /dl (Legal Lim it) 0.05-0.10% or 50-100 m g /dl (under the influence) 0.25% or 250m g /dl or greater (severe intoxication)
Aldolase (ALD)	Adult = 3-8 U /dl (Sibley -Lehninger) 22-50m U /L at 37C .(S Iunits) New born = 12-24 U /dl Pediatric = 6-16 U /dl
Aldosterone (Serum , Urine)	Adult = 1-9 ng /dl (Serum -R IA) Adult = 6-25 ug/24 hrs . (Urine) 5.5-7.2 m m ol/24 hrs. (Urine - S Iunits)

Alkaline Phosphatase (ALP)	Adult = 1.5 -4.5 U/dl(Bodansky) 4-13 U/dl(King-Armstrong) 0.8-2.3 U/ml (Bessey-Lowry) 15-35 U/ml (Shinowar-Jones-Ronhart) 20-90IU/L at30C . (SIunits) Newborn = 40-300 U/L Pediatric = 60-270 U/L 15-30 U/dl (King-Armstrong) 5-14 U/dl(Bodansky) 3.4 -9U/ml (Bessey-Lowry)
Alpha -1 antitrypsin	200-500 mg/dl
ALT	0-40 IU/L
Aminoglycoside Level	Peak = Amikacin = 15-30 ug/ml Gentamicin = 5-10 ug/ml Tobramycin = 5-10 ug/ml Trough = Amikacin <10 ug/ml Gentamicin <2 ug/ml Tobramycin <2ug/ml
Ammonia	Adult = 3.0 -4.5 g/dl 20-120 mg/dl (Diffusion method) 40-80 mg/dl (enzymatic method) 10-40 mg/dl (resin method) 10-35 umol/L (SIunits) Newborn = 90-145 mg/dl Pediatric = 40-80 mg/dl
Amylase (Serum)	Adult = 60-160 U/dl(Somogyi) 110-300 U/dl (SIunits) Pediatric = 80-180 U/dl (Somogyi)
Amylase (Urine)	Adult = 35 -260 U/hr (Somogyi) 260-950 U/24hrs (Somogyi) 6.5-48 U/L (SIunits)
Anion gap	8-12 meq/L (mmol/L)
Antinuclear Antibodies	Adult = Negative
Antistreptolysin O (ASO)	AdultO Negative
Asorbic Acid	0.40-1.5 mg/dl
Aspartate Aminotransferase (AST)	Adult = 4-36 U/ml 5-40U/ml (Frankle) 16-60 U/ml at30C . (Karmen) 8-35 U/lat37C . (SIunits) Newborn = Fourtimes the adult level Pediatric = Same as the adult level
Basophils	Adult = 0.5-10% oftotalWBC 0-0.20 x 10 9/L (SIunits) 30-100 cumm .
Bence Jones Proteins	Negative
Bilirubin direct	0-0.4 mg/dl
Bilirubin, Indirect	Adult = 0.2 -0.8 mg/dl 1.8-17 umol/L (SIunits) Newborn = Same as adult
Bilirubin, Total	Adult = 0.2-1.2 mg/dl 1.8-21 umol/L (SIunit) Newborn 0-1.0 mg/dl 17 -205 umol/L
Bilirubin, Urine	Negative

Bleeding Time	Adult = 1-6 minutes (Ivy) 1-6 minutes (Duke) 3-8 minutes (SI units)
Blood Urea Nitrogen	Adult = 10-20 mg/dl (Male) 8-20 mg/dl (Female) Infant = 5-15 mg/dl Pediatric = 5-20 mg/dl
C3 Complement	55-120 mg/dl
C4 Complement	14-51 mg/dl
C-Reactive Protein	Adult and Pediatric = Negative
Calcium	Adult = 4.5-5.6 m Eeeeq/L 9-11 mg/dl 2.3-2.8 mmol/L (SI units) Newborn = 3.7 -7.0 m Eq/L 7.4-14 mg/dl 1.75 -3 mmol/L (SI units) Child = 4.5-5.8 m Eq/L 8-11.5 mg/dl 2.25-2.88 mmol/L (SI units)
Calcium Channel Blockers	Adult Theraputic = 50-200 ng/ml (Diltiazem) 50-100 ng/ml (Nifedipine) 100-300 n/ml (Verapamil) 0.08-0.3 ug/ml
Carcinoembryonic Antigen (Cea)	Adult = < 2.8ng/mlor<2.8 ug/L
Carotene (Carotenoids)	50-300 ug/dl
Catecholamines (Urine)	Adult = <100ug /24 hours <0.6 umol/24 hours (SI units) 0-15 ug/dl (Random) Infant = <20 ug/dl(24hours) Pediatric (1-5 Years) = <40ug/dl (24hours) (5-15 Years) = <80ug/dl (24hours)
Cerebrospinal Fluid Analysis (CSF)	Adult = Color-clear Pressure-75-180 mm H2O Leukocytes-0-8mm 3 Protein-15-48 mg/dl Glucose-40-80 mg/dlor 2.75-4.4 mmol/L Chloride-120-130 m Eeq/L or120-130 mmol/L Pediatric = Color-clear Pressure-50-100 mm H2O Leukocytes 0-8 mm 3 Protein-15-48 mg/dl Glucose-35-75 mg/dl Chloride-122-128 m Eq/L
Ceruloplasmin	15-60 mg/dl
Chloride	Adult = 95-105 m Eq/L 95-105 mmol/L (SI units) Newborn = 94 -115 m Eq/L Infant = 95-110 m Eq/L 1.7 -8.5 mmol/d (SI units) Pediatric = 98 – 105 m Eq/L 17-34 mmol/d (SI units)
Chloride (Sweat)	Adult = <60m Eq/L Pediatric = <50 m Eq/L

Cholesterol	Adult = 150-200 m g /dl 3-6.5 m m ol /L (S I units) Infant = 70-175 m g /dl Child = 120-250 m g /dl
Cholinesterase	Adult RBC = 0.5-1 U 0.65 -1.3 U (S I units) 6-10 IU /L Plasm a = 3-8 U /m l 0.5-1.3 U (S I units) 8-20 IU /L at 37C . Pediatric = Sam e as adult
Cold Agglutinins	Adult and Pediatric <1 :10 R atio (N egative) Abnorm al <1 :32 R atio (Positive)
Com plem ent Test (C3)	Adult 80-180 m g /dl (M ale) 75-125 m g /dl (Fem ale)
Com plem ent Test (C4)	Adult 15-60 m g /dl (M ale) 15-50 m g /dl (Fem ale)
Com plete B lood Count (CBC)	Hem atocrit - Adult = 40-55% (M ale) 38-44% (Fem ale) N ewborn = 45-65% Infant = 40-50% Child = 30-44% Hem oglobin - Adult = 14-18 g /dl or 2.09 - 2.79 m m ol (M ale) 12-16 g /dl or 1.86 - 2.48 m m ol (Fem ale) N ewborn = 12-20 g /dl Infant = 10-14 g /dl Child = 11-13.5 g /dl RBC 's - Adult = 4.5-6 m illion /L or 4.5-6 x 10 12 /L (M ale) 4.2-5.4 m illion /L or 4.2 - 5.4 x 10 12 /L (Fem ale) N ewborn = 4.4 - 5.8 m illion /L Child = 4.6 - 4.8 m illion /L W BC 's - Adult and Pediatric 4-11 thousand cu.m m . D ifferential = N eutrophils = 55-70% or 1.8 -7.8 x 10 9 /L Lym phocytes = 20-40% or 1.0 - 4.8 x 10 9 /L M onocytes = 2-8 % or 0-0.8 x 10 9 /L Eosinophils = 2-4% or 0-0.45 x 10 9 /L Basophils = 0.5-1% or 0-0.2 x 10 9 /L
Coom bs (D irect)	Adult and Pediatric = N egative
Coom bs (Indirect)	Adult and Pediatric = N egative
Copper	100-200 ug /dl
Corticotropin or Corticotropin Releaseing Factor (CRF)	Adult = 8-10 pg /m l (in AM <80pg /m l)
Cortisol	Adult = 5-25 um g /dl (8-10 AM) 140-635 nm ol /L (S I units) 2.5-12.5 um g /dl (4-6 PM) or 70-318 nm ol /L (S I units) Child = 15-25 um g /dl (8-10AM) 5-10 um g /dl (4-6 PM) 1.9-151 um ol /dl (Free)

Creatine Phosphokinase (CPK)	Adult = 55-165 U/L at 37 C. (Male) S I units 30-130 U/L at 37 C. (Female) S I units 10-80 IU/L Child = 0-65 IU/L at 30 C. (Male) 0-50 IU/L at 30 C. (Female) Newborn = 10-300 IU/L at 30 C.
Isoenzymes	CPK-BB = 0 CPK-MB = 0-8 IU /L CPK-MM = 5-70 IU/L
Creatinine	Adult = 0.60 -1.0 mg /dl 53 -106 um ol/L (S I units) Pediatric = 0.3-0.5 mg/dl (0-6 years) 27-54 um ol/L (S I units) 0.4-1.2 mg/dl (7-15 years) 62 -106 um ol/L (S I units)
Creatine Clearance (Urine)	Adult = 100-200 m l/min 1.7-2.3 m l/s (S I units) Pediatric = 98 -150 m l/min i, (Male) 95 - 125 m l/min (Female)
Cryoglobulins	Adult and Child = Negative
Delta Aminolevulinic Acid (ALA)	<200 ug/dl
Digoxin	Theraputic: Adult = 0.6 - 2ng/m l 0.6 -2nm ol/l (S I units) Infant = 1-3 ng/m l Child = Same as adult level Toxic: Adult = > 2 ng /m l > 2.5 nm ol/L (S I units) Infant = >3.5 ng/m l Child = Same as adult
Estrogens	Adult = 10-30 pg/m l (Male) 50-285 pg/m l (Female -Early Cycle) 100-550 pg/m l (Female -Mid Cycle) 80-425 pg/m l (Female -Late Cycle)
Fasting Blood Sugar(FSB)	Adult = 70-110 mg/dl (Serum or Plasma) 60-100 mg/dl (Blood) Newborn = 30-80 mg/dl Child (1-15 Years) = 60-100 mg/dl
Fecal Fat (Stool)	Adult = <7g/24 hours
Alpha Fetoprotein	<40ug/L
Fibrinogen	Adult = 200-400 mg /dl 2-4 g/dl (S I units) Newborn = 150-300 mg/dl
Folate	1.9 -14 ng/m l
Folic Acid	Adult = 5-25 ng /m l (Bioassay) >2.5 ng /m l (RIA) >166 ng/m l (RBC) Pediatric = Same as adult

Follicle-Stimulating Hormone (FSH)	Adult = 5-48 m UU/24 hours (Urine) 4-25 m IU/ml (SI units - Urine) Postmenopause = >48 m UU/24 hours (Urine) 40-50 m IU/ml (SI Units-Urine) Adult = 4-28 m IU/ml (SI units - Female - Serum) 4-22 m IU/ml (SI Units - Male Serum) Pediatric Prepubertal = <10 m UU/24 hours (Urine) 4-30 m IU/ml (SI units)
Gamma-Glutamyl Transferase (GGT)	Adult = 5-40 IU/L 5-38 U/L at 37 C. (SI units)
Gastric Acid Secretion/Gastric Analysis	Adult = 5-40 m Eq/hr (Stimulated) 5-40 mmol/hr (SI units) 1-5 m Eeq/L/hr (Basal Acid Output-BAO) 5-40 mmol/hr (SI units)
Gastrin	Adult = 40-200 pg/ml
Glucose-6-phosphate dehydrogenase	5-10 IU/g Hb
Glucose Tolerance Test (GTT)	Adult = 70-100 mg/dl (Serum - Fasting) 3.85-6.05 mmol/L (Serum - SI units) <160 mg/dl (Serum - 30 minutes) 5.5-9.35 mmol/L (SI units) <170 mg/dl (Serum - 1hour) 4.95-8.8 mol/L (SI units) <125 mg/dl (Serum - 2 hours) 4.13-6.88 mmol/L (SI units) 70-100 mg/dl (Serum - 3 hours) 3.85-6.05 mmol/L (SI units) Pediatric = More than 6 years old = Same as adult
Haptoglobin (Hp)	Adult = 50-270 mg/dl 0.7-2.9 g/L (SI units) Infant = 0-32 mg/dl Newborn 0-8 mg/dl
Hepatic Antigen (HAA, HBsAg)	Adult and Pediatric = Negative
Human Chorionic Gonadotropin (HCG)	Adult = Positive or Negative (Pregnancy)
Human T Lymphotropic Virus-III (HTLV - III)	Adult or Pediatric = Negative
17 - Hydroxycorticosteroids (17-OHCS)	Adult = 4-13 mg/24 hrs (Male) 3-12 mg/24 hrs (Female) Pediatric = 3.0+1.0m g/m 2/24hours (less than 16 years old)
5 Hydroxyindoleacetic Acid (5-HIAA)	Adult = Negative (Urine - Random) 3-10 mg/24 hours (Urine Quantitative)

Immunoglobins (Ig)	Adult = 900-2100 g/L (Total - SI units)
	     800-1850 g/L (IgG)
	     100-400 g/L (IgA)
	     50-150 g/L (IgM)
	     0.5-2.5 g/L (IgD)
	Newborn = 650-1400 g/L (Total)
	     650-1250 g/L (IgG)
	     0-11 g/L (IgA)
	     5-35g/l (IgM)
	3-5 months = 325 - 700 (Total)
	     275-750 g/L (IgG)
	     5-55 g/L (IgA)
	     15-75 g/L (IgM)
	6-11 months = 225-1200 g/L (Total)
	     200 -1100 g/L (IgG)
	     10-90 g/L (IgA)
	     10-80 g/L (IgM)
	1-3 Years = 700-1600 g/L (Total)
	     650-1300 g/L (IgG)
	     50-200 g/L (IgA)
	     30-120 g/L (IgM)
	4-9 Years = 400 -1550 g/L (Total)
	     300-1400 g/L (IgG)
	     20-175 g/L (IgA)
	     20-100 g/L (IgM)
	10-16 Years = 700 -1600 g/L (Total)
	     550 -1450 g/L (IgG)
	     50-200 g/L (IgA)
	     22-120 g/L (IgM)

Iron (Fe)	Adult = 10-25 um ol/L (SI units) Newborn 100-200 ug/dl Child = 40-100 ug/dl
Iron Binding Capacity (TIBC)	Adult = 250-400 ug/dl 54-64 um ol/L (SI units) Newborn = 60-170 ug/dl Child = 100-350 ug/dl
Ketone Bodies	Adult or Pediatric = Negative

17 Ketosteroids (17KS)	Adult = 7-26 m g/24 hours (Male Urine)
	     5-15 m g/24 hours (Female Urine)
	Geratric = 5-8 m g/24 hours
	Pediatric = < 4m g/24 hours (3-10 Years)
	     13-18 m g/24 hours (Male)
	     3-12 m g/24 hours (Female)

Lactic Dehydrogenase (LDH)	Adult = 150-450 U/m l (W roblew ski-Total) 80-120 U/m l (W alkerUnits) 100-200 IU /L 30-62 U/L at 30 C . (SIunits) LDH 1 = 18-27% or 0.18 - 0.27 (SIunits) LDH 2 = 28-38% or 0.28-0.38 (SIunits) LDH 3 = 18-26% or 0.18-0.26 (SIunits) LDH 4 = 4-9% or 0.04-0.09 (SIunits) LDH 5 = 0-5 % or 0-0.5 (SIunits) N ewborn = 300-1600 IU /L Child = 50-150 IU/L
Lead Lever	Adult = 10-50 ug/dl 0.2um ol/L (SIunits) Child = 10-20 ug/dl (SIunits)
Lidocaine H cl	Adult = 1.1 - 5.6 ug/m l (Theraputic) 5.0-23.4 um ol/L (SIunits) Child = Sam e as adult level
Lipase	Adult = <1.5 U/m l (Cherry-C randall M ethod) 1-21 IU /dl 14-280 m IU/m l 14-280 U/L (SIunits) Infant = 9-105 IU /L at 37 C . Child = 20-136 IU /L at 37 C .
Lithium	Adult = 0.50-1.5 m Eq /L (Theraputic) 0.5-1.5 m m ol/L (SIunits)
Lupus Test	Adult = N egative Child = N egative
Lym phocytes	Adult = 25-40% of total leukocytes 1500-3500 m m 3 1.0-4.8 x 10^9 /L (SIunits) N ewborn = 32%
M agnesium	Adult = 1.5-2.1 m Eq/L 0.7-1.1 m m ol/L (SIunits) Childs = 1.7-2.2 m Eq/L
O ccult B lood	Adult or Pediatric = N egative
O sm olality	Adult = 500-800 m O sm /kg/H_2O (U rine) 500-800 m m ol/kg (SIunits) N ewborn = 100-550 m O sm /kg/H_2O Child = Sam e as adult
Papanicolaou Test (PAP Sm ear)	Adult = C lass I-Absence of Abnorm al C ells C lass II-Abnorm al C ells ; N o M alignancy C lass III-Suggestive of M alignancy C lass IV -Conclusive of M alignancy
PartialThrom boplastin Tim e (PTT, APPT)	Adult = 50-80 Seconds (PTT) 20-40 Seconds (APPT)
Phenylketonuria (PKU)	Pediatric = N egative

Phenytoin	Adult = 10-20 ug/m l (Theraputic) 40-80 um ol/L (S I units) Abnorm al Adult = >20ug /m l (Toxic) >79.2 um ol/L (S I units) Abnorm an Pediatric = > 15-20 ug/m l (Toxic) 55-78 um ol/L (S I units)
Phosphorus (P) /Phosphate (PO 4)	Adult = 0.76 -1.50 m m ol/L (S I untis) 1.7 -2.5 m Eq /L 2.5-4.6 m g/dl Newborn = 3.5 -8.5 m g/dl Infant = 4.5 -6.5 m g /dl Child = 4.5-5.5 m g/dl
Platelet Count	Adult = 150,000 - 400,000 m m 3 0.15-0.5 x 10 12 /L (S I units) Newborn = 150,000 -300,000 m m 3 Child = 175,000-450,000 m m 3
Postprandial B lood Sugar (2hour Postprandial B lood Sugar)	Adult and Child = <138 m g/dl/2 hours (Serum) Adult and Child = <120 m g/dl/2 hours (B lood)
Potasium (K+)	Geriatric = 3.5-5.6 m Eq /L Adult = 3.5-5.0 m Eq /L 3.5-5.0 m m ol/L (S I units) Child = 3.5-4.7 m Eq /L Newborn = 5.0-7.7 m Eq /L
Pregnanediol	Adult = 0.1-1.4 m g/24 hours (M ale) 0-5 um ol/24 hours (S I units) Adult = 0.5-1.5/24 hours (Fem lae - Proliferation) 3-25 um ol/24 hours (S I units) 2-7 m g/24 hours (Luteal) 0.1-1.0 m g/24 hours (Postm enopause)
Pregnanetriol	Adult = 0.4-2.5 m g/24 hours (M ale -Urine) 1.2-7 um ol/24 hours (S I units) 0.5-2 m g/24 hours (Fem ale) 1.5-6 um ol/24 hours (S I units) Infant = 0-0.2 m g/24 hours Child = 0-0.9 m g/24 hours 0-3 um ol/24 hours (S I units)
Protien, Total	Adult = 6-8 g/dl 6-8 g/L (S I units) Newborn = 4.5-7.5 g/dl Infant = 6.0-6.5 g/dl Child = 6.2-8.0 g/dl
Protein, Serum Electrophoresis	Adult = 52-65% or 3.2-5.6 gm /dl (A lbum in) 0.52-0.65 (Fraction -S I units) Child = 4.0-5.8 gm /dl (A lbum in) Adult = 2.5-5.0% or 0.1-0.4 gm /dl (alpha 1) 0.25-0.5 (Fraction S I units) Child = 0.1-0.4 gm /dl (alpha 1) Adult = 7.0-13% or 0.4-1.2 gm /dl (alpha 2) 0.7-0.13 (Fraction S I units) Child = 0.4-1.0gm /dl (alpha 2) Adult = 8.0-14% or 0.5-1.6 gm /dl (beta) 0.8-0.14 (Fractiooon S I units) Child = 0.5-1.0 gm /dl (beta) Adult = 12-22% or 0.5-1.6 gm /dl (gam m a) 0.12-0.22 (Fraction S I units) Child 0.3-1.0 gm /dl (gam m a)

Prothrombin (PT)	Adult or Pediatric = 9-12 Seconds
Radioactive Iodine Uptake Test (RAI)	Adult = 1-13% (2 hours) 2-25% (6 hours) 15-40% (24 hours)
Renin	Adult = 0.5-4.5 ng/ml/hours
Reticulocyte Count	Adult = 0.5-1.5% of all Rbc's 25,000 - 75,000 mm3 Newborn = 2-5% of all RBC's Infant = 0.5-4% of all RBC's Older Child = 0.5-2% of all RBC's
Rheumatoid Factor (RF, RA Factor)	Adult = Negative or less than 1:20 titre
Rubella Titre	Adult = Negative
Salicylate	Adult = <30 mg/dl (Theraputic) > 30 mg/dl (Minor Toxicity) > 50 mg/dl (Major Toxicity) Pediatric > 28 mg/dl (Toxic)
Schilling Test	Adult = > 7%
Sedimentation Rate (ESR)	Adult - Male = 0-17 m/hr (Westergran Method - SI units) 0-7 mm/hr (Cutler Method - SI units) 0-6 mm/hr (Wintrobe Method - SI units) Adult - Female = 0-20 mm/hr (Western Method - SI units) 0-9 mm/hr (Cutler Method - SI units) 0-13 mm/hr (Wintrobe Method - SI units)
Semen Test (Sperm Test)	Adult = Volume 1-5.5 ml 0.0015-0.005/L (SI units) Count 60-175 million/ml 60-175 x 10^9/L (SI units) Motility >70% Mature >0.7 (Fraction - SI units)
Skin Test, Blastomycosis	Adult = Negative
Skin Test, Coccidiodomycosis	Adult = Negative
Skin Test, Histoplasmosis	Adult = Negative
Skin Test, Toxoplasmosis	Adult = Negative
Skin Test, Trichinosis	Adult = Negative
Skin Test, Tuberculosis	Adult = Negative
Sodium (Na+)	Geriatric = 134-147 mEq/L 134-147 mmol/L (SI units) Adult = 136-145 mEq/L 136-145 mmol/L (SI units) Child = 138-145 mEq/L 138-145 mmol/L (SI units) Newborn = 126-166 mEq/L 126-166 mmol/L (SI units)
Specific Gravity, Urine	Adult = 1.005-1.030 Newborn = 1.001-1.020 Child 1.005-1.030

Testosterone	Adult (Male) = 0.3-1 .ug/dl 300-1100 ng/dl 10-42 nm ol/L (S I units) Adult (Female) = 0.04-0.1 ug/dl 30-100 ng/dl 1.1-3.3 nm ol/L (S I units) Child = > 0.1ug/dl (More than 12 years old) >100ng/dl
Theophylline	Theraputic - Adult = 5-20 ug/m l 26-110 um ol/L (S I units) Geriatric = 5-17 ug/m l Infant = 3-10 ug/m l Prem ature Infant = 6-14 ug/m l Child = Sam e as adult levels Toxic - Adult = >20ug/m l >110um ol/L (S I units)
Throm boplastin	Adult and Child = Usually 20-30 seconds
Thyroid - Stim ulating Horm one (TSH)	Adult = 2-5-5 uIU/m l <3ng/m l >10 -3 IU/L (S I units) Newborn and Pediatric = <25uIU/m l
Thyroxine (T4)	Adult = 4.5-11.5 ug/dl (Serum) 6.0-11.5 (Murphy-Pattee) 3.2-7.2 ug/dl (Iodine) 4.0-7.5 ug/dl(Murphy-Pattee) 5-12 ug/dl (R IA) 1-2.4 ng/dl(Free) Newborn = 10-22 ug/dl Infant = 5.5 -16 ug/dl Child 5-13 ug/dl
Triglycerides	Adult = 10-190 m g/dl 0.11-2.11 m m ol/L (S I units) Infant = 4-5 m g/dl Child 10-140 m g/dl
Triiodothyronine Uptake (T3)	Adult = 80-200 ng/dl 25-35% 0.25-0.35 (S I units) Newborn = 90-160 ng/dl Child = 110-185 ng/dl
Uric Acid	Adult Male = 4-8 m g/dl 0.24-0.5 m m ol (S I units) Adult Fem ale = 2.8-6.5 m g/dl 0.16-0.4 m m ol/L (S I units) Pediatric = 2.5-5.5 m gg/dl

Urinalysis	Normal = color – straw to amber Appearance – clear pH – 4.5-7.5 Sp.Gr. – 1.005-1.030 Protein – Negative Glucose – Negative Ketones – Negative RBC's – 1-2 WBC's – 3-4
Urobilinogen	Adult and Child = 0.5 -3.2 mg/dl (Random) 0.3-1.0 U (Ehrlich – 2 hour) 0.05-2.5 mg/24 hours 0.5-4.0 U/24 hours (Ehrlich) 0.1-4.2 um ol/24 hours (SI units)
Vanillylmandelic Acid (VMA)	Adult and Pediatric = 7.6-37.5 u/m ol/24 hours (SI units) 1.5-7.5 mg/24 hours
Venereal Disease Research Laboratory (VDRL)	Adult and Pediatric = Negative

PHARMACOLOGY

PHARMACOLOGY

A) To deliver "x" m g/m in	Amount divided by 60 = m g/cc/m in Volume
B) From A you can determine th cc/hr to run the IV pump	$\dfrac{mg/min}{mg/cc/min}$ = cc/hr on the pump
C) To determine the m g/m in the patient is Receiving	Amount divided by 60 x IV Rate Volume
D) To deliver "x" m cg/m in	Amount x 1000 = m cg/cc/m in Volume 60
E) From D you can determine the cc/hr to run the pump	$\dfrac{mcg/min}{mcg/cc/min}$ = cc/hr to run the pump
F) To determine the m cg/m in the patient is Receiving	Amount x 1000 x IV Rate Volume 60
G) To determine the desired m cg/m in	Desired m cg x kg x 60 mcg /cc
H) To determine the cc/hr to run the pump	m cg x kg x 60 = cc/hr to run the pump m gx1000 Volume
I) To determine the m cg/kg/m in the patient is Receiving	$\dfrac{mg}{Volume}$ x $\dfrac{100}{60}$ x $\dfrac{cc/hr}{kg}$

	DRUG	AMOUNT
Adult Emergency Intravenous Bolus Medications	Atropine	0.50-1.0 m g q5" (Up to 2 m g)
	Epinephrine	0.5-1.0 m g q5"
	Lidocaine	1m g/kg
	Bretylium	5-10 m g/kg q15-30"
	Sodium Bicarbonate	1 m Eq/kg
	Procainamide	10-12 m g/kg
	Calcium Chloride	0.5-1 gram
	Calcium Gluconate	0.5-1 gram
	Verapamil	2.5-10 m g (x2 doses if needed)

Pediatric Em ergency Resuscitation Drugs	Epinephrine	0.01 m g/kg/dose = 0.1 cc/kg of a 1:10,000 solution
	Sodium Bicarbonate	1 m Eq/kg of a 8.4% solution
	Atropine	0.01-0.02 m g/kg/dose
	Calcium Chloride	10-20 m g/kg
	Calcium Gluconate Lidocaine	20/m g/kg
		1 m g/kg
	Bretylium Tosylate	5 m g/kg
	Am rinone	1-3 m g/kg
	Glucose	0.5-1.0
Pediatric Em ergency Infusion Rates	Epinephrine	0.1-1.0 ug/kg/m in
	Dopam ine	2-20 ug/kg/m in
	Dobutam ine	5-20 ug/kg/m in
	Isoproterenol	0.1-1.0 ug/kg/m in
	Lidocaine	20-50 ug/kg/m in

	DRUG	AMOUNT	RATE
Pediatric Infusion Rate M ixtures by W eight (Infuse at 1 m l/kg/hr)	Isoproterenol Epinephrine Dopam ine Dobutam ine	0.6 m g/100 m l 0.6 m g/100 m l 60 m g/100 m l 60 m g/100 m l	0.1 ug/kg/m in 0.1 ug/kg/m in 10 ug/kg/m in 10 ug/kg/m in
Pediatric Infusion Rates M ixtures (Infuse at 1 m l/hr)	Dopam ine/Dobutam ine/Am rinone	15 x W t(kg) = #m g/250m l	1 ug/kg/m in
	Nitroprusside/Nitroglycerine Prostaglandin	1.5 x W t(kg) = #m g/250m l	0.1 ug/kg/m in
	Epinephrine/Isoproterenol/ Norepinephrine	0.15 x W t(kg) = #m g/250m l	0.01 ug/kg/m in

RESPIRATORY

Respiratory

Oxygen Delivery Device	Flow Rate	FiO2
Nasal Cannula	1	24%
	2	28%
	3	32%
	4	36%
	5	40%
	6	44%
Simple Mask	5	40%
	6	45-50%
	8	55-60%
Non-Rebreather	6	55-60%
	8	60-80%
	10	80-90%
	12	90%
	15	90-100%
Partial Rebreather	6	35%
	7	40%
	8	45%
	9	50%
	10	60%
	12	60%
	15	60%
Venturi Mask	Blue - 4 L	24%
	Yellow - 4L	28%
	White - 6L	31%
	Green - 8L	35%
	Pink - 8L	40%

BASIC RESPIRATORY EQUATIONS:	KEY FOR ABBREVIATIONS:
$Vc = RV + Vt + ERV$	CiHe = Initial concentration of helium in the spirometer
	CfHe = Initial concentration of helium in the spirometer
$Vc = IC + ERV$	

TLC = Vc + RV	Vispir = Initial volume of the spirom eter
TLC = IC + FRC	Vc = Vital C apacity
	RV = Inspiratory Reserve Volume
FRC = ERV + RV	VT = Tidal Volume
	ERV = Expiratory Reserve Volume
RV + FRC – ERV	IC = Inspiratory Capacity
FRC = (CiHe –1) (CfHe) X Vispir	TLC = TotalLung Capacity
	RV = Residual Volume
	FRC = Functional Residual Capacity

NORMAL RESPIRATORY VALUES (DEPENDENT ON SIZE)

Parameter	Male	Female
Total Lung Capacity (TLC)	6-7 L	5-6L
Functional Residual Capacity (FRC)	2-3L	2-3L
Residual Value (RV)	1-2L	1-2L
Forced Vital Capicity (FVC)	4L	3L
Forced Vital Capacity at 1 sec. (FEV1)	>3L	>2L
Pulmonary Compliance	<3cm H20 /sec/L	<3cm H20 /sec/L
	<2.5cm H2o/sec/L	<2.5cm H2o/sec/L
Pulmonary Resistance (RL)	0.2L/cm /H20	0.2L/cm /H20
Airway Resistance		
Pulmonary Compliance		

FORMULAS	NORMALS
Arterial 02 Content $CaO_2 = 1.39 \times Hgb \times SaO_2 + 0.0031 \times PaO_2$	18-20 m l/dl
M ixed Venous 0 2 Content $CvO_2 = 1.39 \times Hgb \times SvO_2 = 0.0031 \times PvO_2$	13-16 m l/dl
Arteriovenous 0 2 Content D ifference $avDO_2 = CaO_2 - CvO_2$	4-5.5 m l/dl

Pulmonary Capillary O2 Content $CAO_2 = 1.39 \times Hgb \times SaO_2 + 0.0031 \times PaO_2$	20 ml/dl
Pulmonary Shunt $Qs/Qt = 100 \times CAO_2 - Cao_2 / CAO_2 - CVO_2$	2-8%
Percent Arteriovenous Shunt $Qs/Qt = 100 \times \dfrac{Hgb \times 1.34 \times (1 - \{SaO_2/100\}) + 0.0031\ (PAO_2 - PaO_2)}{Hgb \times 1.34 \times (1 - \{SvO_2/100\}) + 0.0031\ (PAO_2 - PvO_2)}$	3-5%
Oxygen Transport $O_2\ transport = 10 \times CO \times CaO_2$	880-1040 ml/min
Oxygen Consumption $VO_2 = 10 \times CO \times (CaO_2 - CVO_2)$	195-265 ml/min
Oxygen Transport Index $O_2\ Transport\ Index = O_2\ Transport / BSA$	550-650 ml/min/m2
Oxygen Consumption Index $O_2\ Consumption\ Index = VO_2 / BSA$	115-165 ml/min/m2
Oxygen Extraction Ratio $O_2ER = (CaO_2 - CVO_2)/CaO_2$	0.24-0.28
Alveolar Arterial Oxygen Difference $AaDo_2 = PAO_2 - PaO_2$ and $PAO_2 = FiO_2 \times (bp - 47) - PaCo2$	10-65 mm Hg on 100% or 10-15 mm Hg on RA
Minute Volume: Minute Volume = TV x Resp Rate /1000	2.5 - 7 L/min
Compliance: Compliance = $\dfrac{Change\ in\ Volume}{Change\ in\ Pressure}$	25-35 ml/cm H2O
Dead Space: Dead Space = (PaCo2 - PECO2) x TV /PaCo2	145-155 ml
Dead Space / Tidal Volume Ratio $Vd/Vt = \dfrac{PaCo2 - PECO2}{PaCo2}$	0.25-0.40
Alveolar Ventilation Alveolar Vent. (in ml/min) = (TV - Vd) x Resp Rate	4-5 LPM
Alveolar - Arterial Gradient: $AaDO_2 = (FiO_2)(713) - PaO_2 - PaCO_2$	>620 mm Hg
Oxidation Index $\dfrac{Mean\ Airway\ Pressure \times FiO_2 \times 100}{Postductal\ PaO_2}$	>40=Mortality of 80-90% >25-40=Mortality of 50-60%

Alveolar Oxygen Partial Pressure (at sea level and FiO2=0.21)
PAO2=150–(1.2 x PaCO2)

Formula for determining initial peak inspiratory flow settings:
V=(VT x f) X (I + E)

Where :

V=Flow Rate (L/min)
VT=Tidal Volume (Liters)
f=Frequency of Breaths per minute
I=Inspiratory portion of breathing cycle
E=Expiratory portion of breathing cycle

Abbreviations for Formulas:

BP=Barometric Pressure (mm Hg)
FiO2=Inspired Oxygen Fraction
PaCO2=Partial presure of arterial carbon dioxide (mm Hg)
PACO2=Partial presure of alveolar carbon dioxide
PaO2=Partial pressure of arterial oxygen
PAO2=Partial pressure of alveolar oxgen
Hgb=Hemoglobin
CaO2=Arterial oxygen content
CAO2=Alveloar oxygen content
CVO2=Venous oxygen content
SaO2=Oxygen Saturation
PECO2=Partial pressure of expired carbon dioxide

Comparison of the different types of High-Frequency Ventilation (HFV):

PARAMETER	HFPPV	HFJV	HFO
Tidal Volume	3-5 m l/kg	2-5 m l/kg	1-3 m l/kg
Frequency	60-150 Breaths /m in	100-300 Breaths /m in	900-30,000 Oscillations / m in
Inspiratory Time	<0.3 sec	<0.2 sec	N/A

Positive - Pressure Ventilation (PPV) vs. High-Frequency Ventiliation (HFV):

PARAMETER	PPV	HFV
Tidal Volume	>than dead space (10-15 m l/kg)	≥ to dead space (< 5m 1/kg)
Frequency	<30 Breaths /m in	> 60 -3000 Breaths /m in
Inspiratory Time	0.8 -1.2 sec.	< 0.3 sec.

Suction Catherter Sizes :

Weight	Average Age	Size
3-5 kg	Newborn	6 Fr.
5-12 kg	2 Months -2 Years	8 Fr.
12-38 kg	2-11 Years	10 Fr.
38-50 kg	11 Years and up	12 Fr.

Normal Respiratory Rates:

AGE	RATE (per minute)
Premature - 6 Months	40-60
6-12 Months	26-30
1-2 Years	21-25
3-10 Years	20
10 Years and up	12-20

Endotracheal Tube Sizes:

AGE:	INTERNAL TUBE SIZE (mm)
Premature	2.5*
Newborn	3.0*
6 Months	3.5*
18 Months	4.0*
3 Years	4.5*
5 Years	5.0*
6 Years	5.5*
8 Years	6.0*
12 Years	6.5
16 Years (or small adult)	7.0
Small Adult	7.0-8.0
Average Adult	8.0-8.5
Large Adult	8.5-9.0
Very Large Adult	10.0 -11.5

* Cuffless Tube

Oral Airway:

AGE	SIZE
Premature	000
Newborn	00
Infant	0
1-3 Years	1
3-8 Years	2
9-18 Years	3
Medium Adult	4
Large Adult	5-6

Nasopharangeal Airway:

Approximate Body Weight	Size (mm)
<100 Pounds	5-6 (small)
101-150 Pounds	7-8 (medium)
>151 Pounds	9-10 (large)

Suction Pressure Settings:

Age	Wall Setting (mm Hg)	Portable Setting (inches of H2O)
Infant (1 Year)	60-80	3-5
Child (1-8 Years)	80-120	5-10
Adult (Average)	120-150	10-15
Adult (Over 75 Years)	80-120	5-10

HEMODYNAMICS

HEMODYNAMICS

FORMULAS	NORMAL VALUES

Cardiac Output (C.O.)
  C.O. = HR x SV
 	
  *HR - Heart Rate (Beats per Minute)
  *S.V. - Stroke Volume (Milliliters per Beat)
	4-8 Liters /Minute

Stroke Volume (S.V.) S.V. = $\dfrac{C.O. \times 1000}{H.R.}$	60-90 Milliliters /Beat

Cardiac Index (C.I.)
  C.I. = C.O. / B.S.A.
 	
  *C.O. - Cardiac Output (Liters /Minutes)
  *B.S.A. - Body Surface Area (Meters 2)
	2.8 - 4.2 Liters /Minute /M2

Mean Arterial Pressure (MAP) MAP = $\dfrac{(Systolic\ B.P.) + (2 \times Diastolic\ B.P.)}{3}$	80-100 mm Hg
Central Venous Pressure (CVP)	2-6 mm Hg or 4-15 cm H2O
Systemic Vascular Resistance (SVR) SVR = $\dfrac{(MAP-CVP) \times 80}{C.O.}$	770-1500 Dynes - sec /cm 5
Pulmonary Artery Systolic Pressure (PAS)	20-30 mm Hg
Pulmonary Artery Diastolic Pressure (PAD)	10-15 mm Hg

Mean Pulmonary Artery Pressure (MPAP) $MPAP = \dfrac{(PAS) + (2 \times PAD)}{3}$	15-20 mm Hg
Pulmonary Capillary Wedge Pressure (PCWP)	8-12 mm Hg
Pulmonary Vascular Resistance (PVR) $PVR = \dfrac{(MPAP - PCWP) \times 80}{C.O.}$	45-120 Dynes /sec /cm 5

HEMODYNAMICS - CON'T.

FORMULAS	NORMAL VALUES
Stroke Volume Index (SVI) $SVI = \dfrac{CI \times 1000}{HR.}$	33-47 cc /beat /m 2
Left Ventricular Stroke Work Index (LVSWI) $LVSWI = SVI (MAP - PCWP) \times 0.0136$	35 - 85 g /m 2 /beat
Right Ventricular Stroke Work Index (RVSWI) $RVSWI = SVI (PAM - CVP) \times 0.0136$	7-12 g /m 2 /beat
Stroke Index (SI) $SI = SV /BSA$	41-51 ml/m 2
Systemic Vascular Resistance Index (SVRI) $SVRI = SVR \times BSA$	1970 - 2390 Dynes -sec /cm 5 -m 2
Pulmonary Vascular Resistance Index (PVRI) $PVRI + PVR \times BSA$	225 - 315 Dynes -sec /cm 5 -m 2

Left Cardiac Work (LCW) LCW = C.O. x MAP x 0.0136	5.4 – 8.8 kg -m
Left Cardiac Work Index (LCW I) LCW I= LCW /BSA	3.4 -4.2 kg -m /m 2

NORMAL HEMOGLOBIN, BLOOD PRESSURE, and HEART RATES in CHILDREN

Age	Hemoglobin	Blood Pressure (Mean)	Heart Rate
Premature	18-22 gm /dl	75/50	125 +/- 50
Term Newborn	18-22	80/46	140 +/- 50
2 Weeks	17	83/49	140 +/- 50
1-6 Months	10	96/65	130 +/- 45
6-12 Months	10-11	99/65	115 +/- 40
1-2 Years	10-12	100/60	110 +/- 40
3-5 Years	12.5 -13	100/60	105 +/- 35
8-10 Years	13-14	110/60	95 +/- 30
12-16 Years	14-15	120/65	82 +/- 25

NORMAL BLOOD PRESSURES (AVERGES)

AGE	MEAN SYSTOLIC	MEAN DIASTOLIC
Newborn	80 +/- 16	46 +/- 16
6 Months -1 Year	89 +/- 29	60 +/- 10
1 Year	96 +/- 30	66 +/- 25
2 Years	99 +/- 25	64 +/- 25
3 Years	100 +/- 25	67 +/- 23

4 Years	99 +/- 20	65 +/- 20
5-6 Years	94 +/- 14	55 +/- 9
6-7 Years	100 +/- 15	56 +/- 8
7-8 Years	102 +/- 15	56 +/- 8
8-9 Years	105 +/- 16	57 +/- 9
9-10 Years	107 +/- 16	57 +/- 9

Normal Blood Flow in the Newborn = (1-35 hours)

Systemic - 2.6 L / min / m2 (Average)
1.5 - 4.1 L / min / m2 (Range)

Pulmonary - 3.0 L / min / m2 (Average)
1.7 - 5.3 L / min / m2

NORMAL PRESSURES OF THE HEART

Pressures	Range (in m m Hg)
Right Atrium (Mean) a wave z point c wave x wave v wave y wave	1-5 2.5-7 1.5-5 1.5-6 0-5 2-7.5 0-6
Right Ventricle Peak Systolic End diastolic	17-32 1-7
Pulmonary Artery (Mean) Peak Systolic End Diastolic	9-19 17-32 4-13

Pulmonary Artery Wedge	4.5-13

Left Atrium (Mean)
  a wave
  z point
  v wave
	2-12
	4-16
	1-13
	6-21

Left Ventricle
  Peak Systolic
  End Diastolic
	90-140
	5-12

CARDIOVASCULAR PERFUSION

CARDIOVASCULAR PERFUSION

TUBING SIZES:

BSA (m 2)	Arterial Line	Venous Line
0-0.5	1/4"	1/4"
0.5-0.85	1/4"	3/8"
0.85-1.5	3/8"	3/8"
1.5 and up	3/8"	1/2"

Arterial and Venous Cannulae Sizes:

BSA (m 2)	Arterial (French)	SVC (mm)	IVC (mm)
0-0.25	10-12	12	16
0.26-0.35	10-12	14	18
0.36-0.45	10-12	16	20
0.46-0.55	14-16	18	22
0.56-0.70	14-16	20	24
0.71-0.85	14-16	22	26
0.86-1.0	18-20	24	28
1.01-1.25	18-20	26	30
1.26-1.45	18-20	28	32
1.46-1.70	18-20	30	34
1.71-1.95	24	32	36
1.95 and greater	26-28	34	38

Pressure Gradients Across Arterial Cannulae (mm Hg)

	FLOW (LITERS per MIN)										
Size (FR)	0.5	1	1.5	2	2.5	3	3.5	4	4.5	5	5.5
10	55	115	185								
12	40	75	135	185							
14	30	55	100	135	190						
16		30	50	65	90	120	145				
18			35	45	50	70	90	100	120	140	
20				35	45	60	70	80	95	110	125
22					40	45	60	65	75	85	95
24					35	40	50	55	65	75	85

Venous Cannulae Drainage:

SIZE (French)	Venous Line Size	Drainage (ml/min)
24	1/4"	1250
26	1/4"	1400
28	1/4"	1750
30	1/4"	2200
32	3/8"	3000
34	3/8"	3200
36	3/8"	3400
38	3/8"	3600
40	1/2"	4000

Recommended Estimated Blood Flows:

Weight (kg)	Flow (cc/kg)
0-3	150-200
3-10	125-150
11-15	100
16-25	90
26-35	80
>35	70

Estimated Blood Volume:

Weight (kg)	Blood Volume (ml/kg)
0-10	80
10-20	75
20-30	70
30-40	65
>40	60

Arterial and Venous Cannulas Sizes and Flow Rates:

BSA	VENOUS		ARTERIAL		FLOW (L/min)
	Double	2 Stage	French	Metric	
1.0	24x26	40x32	18	6.5	2.4
1.1	24x26	40x32	18	6.5	2.6
1.15	24x26	40x32	18	6.5	2.8
1.2	24x26	40x32	18	6.5	2.9
1.3	26x28	40x32	18	6.5	3.1
1.4	26x28	40x32	18	6.5	3.4
1.5	28x30	40x32	20	6.5	3.6
1.6	28x30	40x32	20	6.5	3.8
1.7	30x32	40x32	20	6.5	4.1
1.8	30x32	40x32	20	6.5	4.3
1.9	32x34	40x32	22	8.0	4.6
2.0	32x34	46x34	22	8.0	4.8
2.1	34x36	46x34	22	8.0	5.0
2.2	34x36	46x34	24	8.0	5.3
2.3	36x36	46x34	24	8.0	5.5
2.4	36x36	46x34	24	8.0	5.8
2.5	36x36	46x34	24	8.0	6.0
2.6	36x36	46x34	24	8.0	6.2

Tubing Fluid Volumes:

Size	Volume (ml/ft)
1/2"	39
3/8"	22
1/4"	10
3/16"	5

Arterial Cannula Size Conversion:

French	Millimeters	Inches
2	.67	0.026
4	1.3	0.05
6	2.0	0.08
8	2.7	0.1
10	3.3	0.13
12	4.0	0.16
14	4.7	0.18
16	5.3	0.2
18	6.0	0.23
20	6.7	0.26
22	7.3	0.28
24	8.0	0.31
26	8.7	0.34
28	9.3	0.36
30	10	0.39
32	10.7	0.42

Circulatory Arrest Times:

Patient Temperature (C)	Oxygen Consumption	Duration (Minutes)
37	100%	4-5
29	50%	8-10
22	25%	16-20
16	12%	32-40
10	6%	64-80

Types of Hypothermia:

Type	Temperature (C)	Temperature (F)
Mild	32-37	89.6-98.6
Moderate	28-32	82.4-89.6
Deep	18-28	64.4-82.4
Profound	0-18	32-64.4

Body Surface Area Calculations:

$$BSA = \frac{(Ht.\ in\ cm\ ) \times (Wt.\ in\ kg)}{3600}$$

$$BSA = \frac{(Ht.\ in\ inches) \times (Wt.\ in\ Pounds)}{3131}$$

DUBOIS FORMULA
$$BSA = \frac{(Wt\ in\ kg^{0.425}) \times (Ht\ in\ cm^{0.725}) \times 71.84}{10,000}$$

BOYD FORMULA
$$BSA = \frac{3.207 \times (Ht\ in\ cm^{0.3}) \times (Wt.\ in\ kg \times 1000)^{0.7295\ -\ 0.0188\ log\ (Wt\ in\ kg\ x\ 1000)}}{10,000}$$

Hemodilution Calculations:

- Patient Blood Volume = Patient Wt. (kg) x 70
- System Volume = Prime Volume + Patient Blood Volume
- Red Cell Volume = Patient Blood Volume x Pre op Hct
- On pump Hct = Red Cell Volume / System Volume
- Estimated Hct on pump = (Wt in kg) x Hct / (Wt in kg) + 50

Excessive Chest Tube Drainage:

Pediatric	> 3 m l/kg/hr
Adult	>100 m l/hr

Circulatory Arrest Durgs:

1. Barbituate - (ie.Thiopental)	9-10 m g/kg
2. Corticosteroids - (ie.Methylprednisolone)	30 m g/kg
3. Mannitol	0.25 gm /kg

MISCELLANEOUS

MISCELLANEOUS

RENAL:

	Calculations
Creatinine Clearance=	$\dfrac{UV}{PT}$
Creatinine Clearance (m l/m in/m 2)=	(Ucreat/Screat) x (UrVol/1440) x 1.73/BSA
Anion Gap -	Na+ - HCO3 + Cl-
Osmolality (serum)=	$2 Na (m Eq/L) + \dfrac{BUN (m g/dl)}{2.8} + \dfrac{glucose (m g/dl)}{18}$
HCO3 Deficit=	Body Weight (kg) x 0.4 (Desired HCO3 - Observed HCO3)
Glomerular Filtration Rate =	$\dfrac{U cr x V}{P cr}$
Renal Plasma Flow =	$\dfrac{U pah x V}{P pah}$
Urinary Sodium Excretion (m Eq/day) =	UrNa x UrVol/1000
Urinary Potassium Excertion (m Eq/day) =	UrK x UrVol/1000
Urine Sodium /Potassium Ratio =	UrNa /UrK
Fractional Excretion of Sodium =	UrNa/SerNa) x (Screat/Ucreat) x 100
Osmolar Clearance =	(UrOsm /PDsm) x UrVol
Free Water Clearance (m l/day) =	UrVol- Cosm
Nonsaline Loss =	UrVol- (UrVol x UrNa /140)
BUN /Creatinine Ratio =	BUN /Screat
Urine Serum Creatinine Ratio =	Ucreat /Screat
Urine Plasma Osmolarity Ratio =	UrOsm /PDsm

PROGNOSTIC INDICES:

Peel Index	
1. Age and Sex:	• Men - 54 & under = 0
	55-59 = 1
	60-64 = 2
	65 or > = 3
	• Women - 64 & under = 2
	65 or > = 3

2. Previous history of coronary disease:	• Previous myocardial infarction = 5 • Other cardiovascular disease or history of dyspnea on exertion = 3 • Previous angina = 1 • No cardiovascular disease = 0				
3. Shock:	• absent = 0 • mild or transient = 1 • moderate (present on admit but resolving w/rest & sedation) = 5 • severe and persistent = 7				
4. Left Ventricular Failure:	• Absent = 0 • Basilar Rales = 1 • Dyspnea at rest, pulmonary edema, orthopnea, S3, hepatomegaly, elevated jugular venous pressure or peripheral edema = 4				
5. ECG:	• Normal QRS (ST-T changes only) = 2 • QR complexes = 3 • QS complexes or bundle branch block = 4				
6. Rhythm:	• NSR = 0 • Atrial Fibrillation or Flutter, PAT, frequent PVC's, nodal rhythm, heart block = 4				
Peel Mortality Table:					
SCORE	1-8	9-12	13-16	17-20	21-28
MORTALITY	2.5%	12.5%	23.7%	53.4%	88.5%

Norris Index		
Factor	X	Y

1. Age (yr) - <50
      -50-59
      -60-69
      -70-79
      -80-89
	• 0.2
	• 0.4
	• 0.6
	• 0.8
	• 1.0
		•
		•
		• 3.9
		•
		•

2. Position of Infarct:
  -Anterior transmural
  -Left bundle branch block
  -Inferior &/or posterior transmural
  -Anterior subendocardial
  -Inferior &/or posterior subendocardial
	• 1.0
	• 1.0
	• 0.7
	• 0.3
	• 0.3
		•
		•
		• 2.8
		•
		•

3. Admission Systemic Blood Pressure (mm Hg):
  -<55
  -55-64
  -65-74
  -75-84
  -85-94
  -95-104
  -105-114
  -115-124
  ->125
	• 10.
	• 0.7
	• 0.6
	• 0.5
	• 0.4
	• 0.3
	• 0.2
	• 0.1
	• 0
		•
		•
		•
		• 10.0
		•
		•
		•
		•

4. Heart Size (AP upright taken @ 5 feet) :		
- Normal	• 0	
- Venous Congestion	• 0.3	
- Interstitial Edema	• 0.6	• 1.5
- Pulmonary Edema	• 1.0	
5. Previous history of angina & /or infarction:		
- No Ischemia	• 0	• 0.4
- Previous angina or infarction	• 1.0	

Norris Mortality Table :						
Score	<4	4-5	6-7	8-9	10-11	12
Mortality	3%	8%	22%	40%	65%	78%

Author's Bio

After receiving a Baccalaureate in Nursing, the author continued his career in the field of Cardiovascular Perfusion. The author continued his education graduating from Nova Southeastern University in 1998 with a Master's degree in Health Services Administration. The author and his wife have two children ages two and four.

0-595-21503-3